COMMUNITY ASSESSMENT

COMMUNITY ASSESSMENT

Guidelines for developing countries

DOUGLAS STOCKMAN

INTERMEDIATE TECHNOLOGY PUBLICATIONS 1994

Intermediate Technology Publications Ltd,
103–105 Southampton Row, London WC1B 4HH, UK.

© Douglas Stockman 1994

ISBN 1 85339 224 3

Printed by SRP, Exeter

Table of Contents

Preface	vii
Chapter 1 Introduction	1
Chapter 2 First steps to community assessment	5
The need for assessment	5
Working with community leaders	7
Where to start	8
Observation methods	10
Chapter 3 Basic demographics	13
Population density	14
Fertility rate and family composition	15
Socioeconomic indicators	19
Chapter 4 Water and sanitation	25
Water quality	25
Water quantity	27
Human waste disposal	28
Disease transmission by water contact	29
Water-related diseases	30
Chapter 5 Food - preparation and nutrition	35
Maternal effects on child nutrition	35
Child nutrition	37
Food availability - family level	39
The cooking facility and cooking methods	40
Food selection	43

Chapter 6 Food - agriculture 49

    Food source and food availability 49

    Factors limiting crop yield 51
        1.   Seed variety 51
        2.   Irrigation 52
        3.   Fertilizer use 53
        4.   Land management 57
        5.   Harvesting and storage 58

Chapter 7 Identification of community resources 63

    People 63
        1.   Leaders 63
        2.   Skilled workers 63
        3.   Literate people 64
        4.   Community members 64
        5.   Traditional healers 64

    Raw Materials 65
        1.   Building materials 65

    Transportation methods 67
        1.   Cars and trucks 67
        2.   Human-powered transportation 68
        3.   Animal-powered transportation 68
        4.   Water transportation 69

    Alternative energy sources 69
        1.   Humans and animals 69
        2.   Electricity and fossil fuels 70
        3.   Natural energy sources 70

    Monetary and material resources 72

    Outside resources 74
        1.   Money 74
        2.   Personnel 75
        3.   Books and educational materials 76

Chapter 8 Health, health care and endemic diseases 79

    Health care availability 79
        1.   Barriers to health care 81
        2.   Health facility services 84
        3.   Essential medicines 85
        4.   Vertical programmes 87

At-risk groups 88
1. Women 88
2. Children 91
3. The elderly 100
4. Other at-risk groups 101

Common and endemic diseases 103
1. Disease prevalence and identification 104
2. Detection of onchocerciasis 107
3. Nightblindness - a screening tool for xerophthalmia 109
4. Haematuria and proteinuria as an indicator of schistosomiasis 110
5. Estimating malaria prevalence 111

Chapter 9   Rapid epidemiological assessment 123

Cluster sampling 123

Verbal autopsy 125

Estimating maternal mortality by the sisterhood method 127

Questionnaires aimed at key informants 130

REA summary 133

Appendices

1. International agricultural research centres 135
2. REA equations 136
3. Health survey guidelines 137
4. Sources for published materials pertaining to international health 138

Index 139

Preface

The writing of this book resulted from a terrible tragedy. I was living in a small rural Liberian village when the Liberian civil war of 1989 forced me to return to the USA. Had it not been for the civil war I would have remained too busy to compile this book. On arrival in the USA, I busied myself reading all that I could about primary health care and rural development. I wanted to compare my observations and solutions with those of others. I also needed to catch up on the vast amounts of research being done in developing countries. As with most other resources, access to professional journals and books is very limited in developing countries. Much of what I had observed corresponded to the observations of others.

Every health care project has strengths and weaknesses. Drawing on personal experience, relevant literature and observation of other health care projects, I noted a few weaknesses which occurred with great regularity. Many projects focussed too narrowly on one or two problems. Ill health results from many interrelated factors. Unless a health care worker sees the big picture, the impact of interventions will be limited. The concepts of primary health care and community health address this shortcoming by encompassing many disciplines.

Another shortcoming is that interventions and introduced technologies are often inappropriate to the situation. Most communities cannot afford the interventions. Significant progress has been made, but many interventions are still beyond the level that most communities can maintain. This is particularly true in rural areas. I suspect most government officials and people from Northern countries cannot comprehend the level of poverty at which most rural inhabitants live. Health care workers must structure interventions within the confines of rural poverty. This may mean compromising quality and quantity. The end result is a partially functioning method rather than a non-functioning one.

A third shortcoming is that external support for interventions is often short-lived. The expectation that a one or two year project is adequate to permanently alter (hopefully, for the better) peoples' lives may be erroneous. A generation of external intervention is probably a more reasonable period. Care must be exercised to avoid dependence on external support. This often requires that the project keep interventions simple and affordable. Education must be the cornerstone of intervention. Community members must be trained to perform an increasing number of jobs that the health care worker performs. The hope is that the health care worker will not be needed after time.

The most significant shortcoming results from inadequate community support for health interventions. Getting that support requires great effort. The health care worker must develop a good rapport with community members, and must be a better listener than a director. Ideally, the health care worker should live in the area and become a member of the community. Sustainability depends on community support, from project conception to maintenance of interventions.

This book was written with these thoughts in mind. Many points may seem simplistic, but simplicity is often the most appropriate approach. A simple but functional method should always be used before a more complex, but attention-getting one. A health care worker must listen to community concerns. Community members have insights to problems and solutions that the health worker lacks. Interventions must be structured within the confines of community resources. Finally, the interrelatedness of causes of ill health cannot be ignored. Remembering these points during the formulation of interventions will lead to simple but sustainable solutions.

This book uses a qualitative approach to community assessment. It is meant for the rural health care worker who is too busy caring for patients to implement a rigorous epidemiological study. It discusses common contributors to ill health. It is hoped that a health care worker can use this information to assess quickly the impact of common problems on health. Most clinicians working in developing countries gain an appreciation for common health problems after spending significant time in the community. Hopefully, this text will expedite that process.

This is an introductory text. It does not purport to be complete. Rather, it introduces some basic concepts using a primary health care approach. It is meant to stimulate further study and innovation. It also provides examples of rapid epidemiological assessment (REA) for those who want a rapid but accurate quantitative assessment.

Douglas Stockman

Chapter 1

Introduction

When one realizes the plight of the majority of the world's inhabitants, it becomes obvious that something needs to be done. Eighty percent of the world's population resides in developing countries in abject poverty with little hope for improvement. The statistics are appalling. Even more shocking is the personal observation of human beings suffering and dying from preventable and easily treatable illnesses. For improvement to occur, the problems and their causes must be identified. Once ascertained, appropriate solutions can be formulated and implemented. Community assessment involves identifying problems at the community level which adversely affect health.

Individual communities in less developed countries differ in many ways, but their health problems are strikingly similar. Members of the World Health Organization (WHO) attending the conference in Alma Ata, USSR in 1978 identified eight problems that were major contributors to ill health for people living in low-income countries [1]. The members thought that even though communities differed significantly in culture and appearance, the causes of ill health were remarkably similar. A framework was needed to address these common risk factors.

At the 1978 Alma Ata Conference the concept of primary health care (PHC) was adopted as the preferred method to combat these common health risks to the world's inhabitants. PHC is based on a concept of preventive medicine and requires the full participation of community members. It is the method used to discover the community-specific causes of these eight common problems, as well as the instrument for change. Table 1.1 lists these problems.

Each point in Table 1.1 is a major contributor to ill health. Addressing and improving each of these will lead to wellness for the recipients of the interventions. Some of the points go beyond what Western medical training deems health-related problems. Non-health factors like agriculture and water supply contribute to malnutrition and diarrhoea. If the health care worker treats the illness, but does nothing to correct the underlying cause, the illness will recur. Western-trained health care professionals need to expand their definition of medicine to include many disciplines like agriculture and water supply which impinge upon health. In this way,

Table 1.1
WHO-identified health priorities

Inadequate health education
Inadequate food supply and poor nutrition
Unsafe water and inadequate basic sanitation
Inadequate maternal and child health
Inadequate family planning
Incomplete immunizations
Uncontrolled endemic diseases
Scarcity of essential drugs

medical professionals can best achieve their goal of improving the health of their patients.

The eight points listed in Table 1.1 guide health care workers towards uncovering the problems that adversely affect health, but they do not identify the community-specific causes for those problems. Community assessment refers to a community-specific evaluation to determine the problems which adversely affect health. In addition, the assessment identifies available resources which can then be used to combat those problems.

Community assessment should be viewed as a screening tool which will guide interventions. If a community is assessed but nothing is done with the information, the question of why valuable resources were wasted must be raised. It is similar to obtaining Pap smears but then not intervening when an abnormal result is obtained. If resources are to be spent in assessing a community, then an intervention plan must also be in place at the start of the investigation.

Functional definition of community

A community is generally defined as a group of people with common beliefs, language and culture. In many instances village or tribal boundaries can delineate a community. In other instances this relationship is inaccurate. If a family or a group of families moves from their tribe and takes up residence in another tribe's village, the recent immigrants should not be considered as part of the community. Even though they live inside the village's boundaries, they may function as a separate community.

Figure 1.1
Clinical diagnosis and community diagnosis compared

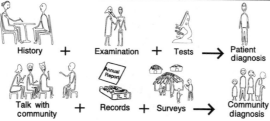

Source: Modified from J. P. Vaughan and R. H. Morrow, (1989). *Manual of Epidemiology for District Health Management*, WHO, Geneva.

The assessment of a community is similar to the evaluation of an ill patient. In the evaluation of a patient a health care worker will obtain a history, perform a physical examination, collect laboratory information, arrive at a diagnosis and recommend treatment. The assessment of a community depends on the same steps. The health care worker will obtain information from community members regarding problems faced by the community, collect information about the community from various sources, perform surveys or evaluations to elucidate the problems further, reach a community diagnosis and recommend possible interventions or treatments (Figure 1.1). In this case the community is the patient and individuals in the community are like organs of a human patient [2].

There are many ways to evaluate a community (Table 1.2). This can vary from an aerial survey of the number of dwellings in a community to a well-controlled experimental study of specific problems within the community. Whatever study method is selected, time must be spent in the community.

Table 1.2
Methods to study communities

Literature review
Direct observation and unstructured
    interviews
Semi-structured interviews:
    key informants
    focus groups
    household interviews
Surveys
Controlled experimental studies

The casual observation of a community can identify factors which adversely affect the health of the community. This level of assessment may be all that is necessary or possible in some situations. Even when a well-controlled epidemiological study is planned, the first step in the design is to observe the community and assess its problems and resources in a non-experimental fashion.

This book addresses the initial observation. It highlights factors which are common contributors to ill health and lays the foundation for further study of the community. The last chapter introduces the concept of rapid epidemiological assessment and offers examples.

References

1. Alma-Ata 1978: Primary Health Care. Geneva, WHO, 1978 (Health for All Series, No. 1).
2. Vaughan J. P., Morrow R. H., (1989). *Manual of Epidemiology for District Health Management*, WHO.

Chapter 2

First steps to community assessment

The need for assessment

Before an assessment is initiated, the community should express a desire for evaluation. People in almost any community will perceive problems and will be interested in assessment of the magnitude of the problems. Whenever a community invites a health care worker to their area, an effort should be made to assess the health problems.

A main point in the WHO's PHC initiative is for community members to participate fully in all activities which affect them. Since the community and its members are the beneficiaries and the driving force behind interventions, it is imperative that all initiatives have community support. Unless community members are actively involved in evaluation, their participation in the improvement process will be negligible [1-3].

Community members must be asked about their perception of community problems (Table 2.1). Health care workers often display significant bias when selecting people to interview. A common mistake is to select only village chiefs and important men. These people generally have the best

Table 2.1 Example list of community member concerns	
Village chiefs, elders and important men	
New village meeting hall	Short-wave transceiver
Tractor to work land	New school
Hospital	Jobs
Isolated villagers	
Truck for transportation	Well for water
Rice	New clothes
Machetes	Medical clinic
Women	
New clothes	Charcoal stove
Transistor radio	Well for water
Mill for grinding foodstuffs	Food for the children
Medicines	

access to resources and therefore have the least need for intervention. Although it is appropriate to meet with leaders first, less visible community members such as women and other at-risk groups must also be identified and interviewed.

Another common selection bias is to visit only easily accessible villages. Again, these people will in general have better access to resources and less need for intervention than their isolated counterparts. For assessment to be accurate and intervention to be successful, perceived problems in the most isolated villages must be revealed. This often requires long walks over difficult terrain. Related to this geographical bias is seasonal bias. Many studies are performed only during the dry season. This is unfortunate because disease prevalence increases during the rainy season.

Significant effort is required to assess the health care needs of isolated community members. Because they often have the greatest health problems, ignoring them defeats the purpose of assessment. During the identification of a representative cross-section of the community, members should be asked to classify perceived problems from the most important to the least important.

Once a list of community concerns is obtained, the health care worker needs to ask difficult questions in order to prioritize the list (Table 2.2). These questions are best answered after the community is surveyed. The process of identifying areas for intervention is always a dynamic one. Problems initially perceived as critical become secondary as new information clarifies the actual determinants of ill health.

Discrepancies will exist between what the community health worker and community members perceive as the most pressing issues. Some level of consensus must be reached. This can result from answering the questions in Table 2.2. For example, the resources may not be available to build a

---

Table 2.2
Questions to refine community concerns

Which are the most serious problems?
Which problems offer the greatest benefits once corrected?
Which problems can be addressed given the available resources?
Which problems are of greatest concern to community members?

Source: WHO, (1988). *Education for Health*, pp.180-185.

new town hall or school. Less costly interventions may address numerous other community concerns.

The problems identified by community members can help focus the fieldworker's assessment. In Table 2.1, community members listed the provision of food, health care, water and cooking facilities as problems. Further observation of these problems may reveal the significant impact each one has on the health of the community. This can address the major objectives of community assessment which are to identify prevalent problems, decide which of these problems are amenable to change, identify readily available resources and, finally, to target which problems can best be addressed with these resources.

If successful intervention is to occur, good relations with community members must be maintained. All community members may not agree with proposed interventions, but good will and understanding need to exist. It is helpful to point out that all problems cannot be addressed at once and that priorities need to be made. Once the most blatant problems are corrected, then other issues may become the area of focus. It is imperative to avoid promising that these secondary concerns will receive attention because the situation may not allow for their resolution.

Working with community leaders

Whenever a health care worker visits a community for the first time, the worker should meet with the recognized leader. It is appropriate in many cultures to ask permission of the leader to visit the community and to interact with its members. Even when invited into the community by non-leader community members, it is wise to meet with the leaders and thank them for their hospitality. Appropriate respect must be shown. This will greatly facilitate further work in the community and will make the leaders more accepting of a health survey.

Within every culture specific rules exist regarding appropriate interaction with leaders. A community member or a health worker who has lived in the area can suggest the best way to approach the leaders. One universal concept, however, is to avoid arrogance. Avoid suggesting that the health care worker has so much to offer that the worker will make all the difference. This approach not only distances most people, it also sets the health care worker up for failure.

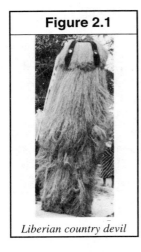

Figure 2.1

Liberian country devil

It must be remembered that the identified leader may not be the most influential leader of the community. Other community members may actually make the important decisions. The identified leader's role may be as a ceremonial figurehead or to deal with minor daily problems. An example of this is when a town chief is the identified leader, but all major decisions are made by the secret society leader or country devil (witch doctor) (Figure 2.2).

In south-east Liberia there are two separate ruling groups in each community. One group consists of the labelled leaders such as the town chief who holds a government position. His job is to enforce governmental policy and uphold Western-style law. The second group of leaders is not easily identified, but constitutes a more powerful governing force in the community's daily life. These leaders are members of the local secret society which is usually headed by the country devil. The country devil controls the spirit world which, in an animist society, controls the happenings of daily life. Therefore, the secret society leaders have greater control over most members of the community. Accessing this leader will be difficult, but successful interventions may depend on the wishes of the invisible leader.

The first meeting with the recognized leader will have a bearing on the willingness of the leader to accept any health survey or visit by a health worker. Good rapport with the leader will increase the chance of access to the community. When the health survey outline is presented to the leaders, it is best to present the concept as a way of helping the health worker learn. This is a true statement and it elevates the leader to a position in which the leader can help the health worker. This will maintain the prestige of the leader in the community and will increase the likelihood that the proposal will be accepted. Possible benefits which may result from the assessment should be mentioned, but care must be taken to offer no more than can be delivered.

Where to start

Community assessment should begin before arrival at the project site. Valuable information exists in the published literature on communities similar to the selected population. Whenever possible, published data should be used to answer questions a new survey was meant to answer. In this way, valuable resources are not wasted gathering information that is currently available. Since many studies are not published, the health care worker has to be creative in locating existing information.

Many sources of relevant published literature exist. Table 2.3 lists examples of these. The advent of computerized databases allows for rapid literature searches. This eases the process of information acquisition. In addition to formal medical databases, anthropological, agricultural and economics databases should be searched. They can provide a flavour for the customs, social structure, political environment and economy of the area. Basic statistics are available for most developing countries. These may be inaccurate, but they are a starting point. Even poorly-collected data can be useful when interpreted with that in mind.

General information regarding the survey site can be found in national and international reports. The WHO and the United Nations Children's Fund (UNICEF) have many reports, both published and unpublished, that can be obtained. Many national agencies like the United States Agency for International Development (USAID) and the European Economic Community (EC) have large ongoing projects in many parts of the developing world. When gathering information from large agencies, it is best to call or write. One cannot rely solely on published reports since much of their information is not distributed to the general public.

The ministry of health of the target country may have statistics about the entire country as well as the survey region. The ministry may also provide

Table 2.3
Sources for statistics

Journals	**PVO/NGO**
Books	Pathfinder Fund
World Health Statistics Quarterly	World Vision
The State of the World's Children	WASH
United Nations Population Division	PAX World, etc.
Demographic Yearbook	**Agency reports**
Demographic and Health Surveys	USAID
Institute for Resource Development	CDC
University projects	EC
Ministry of health in target country	UNICEF
Local hospitals	Peace Corps

the names of agencies which have completed similar studies. Unfortunately, some ministries of health are understaffed and have too small a budget to offer assistance. Expand the search to other ministries such as agriculture, rural development, education and sanitation.

Other intra-country sources of information are government and missionary hospitals. Most hospitals keep registries which may be available for use by non-hospital health workers. It must be remembered that hospital statistics can present a skewed view of the population since a disproportionate number of patients come from the wealthy educated class. If a local clinic exists in the project site, it can be a useful source of information.

Private voluntary organizations (PVOs) and non-governmental organizations (NGOs) have played a major role in the delivery of health care in less developed countries (LDCs). They often provide useful information. Although they expend most of their energies in providing services, they do spend some time researching the population.

Universities and schools of public health, both domestic and abroad, have health projects in developing countries. They may be helpful in delineating common health problems. Again, the ministry of health can direct the health care worker to these valuable resources.

One overlooked source of information is that obtained from those who have lived in the project site. Peace Corps and missionary hospital volunteers are numerous and may presently live in your area. Locating such people may depend on word-of-mouth information since many agencies refuse to release personal data about their members. If located, they can provide a personal view of the problems present in the study area. Since personal observations can be biased, the source of the information must be considered when weighing its applicability.

Observation methods

Simple observation is a required step in community assessment. This applies to both intervention-directed studies and research-directed studies. Simple observation, which includes talking with community members, provides information to direct a comprehensive assessment. A poorly performed initial examination can result in a misdirected community assessment. The end result may be useless information and wasted resources.

In some cases, simple observation provides enough information to direct interventions. Because of this, casual community assessment should occur every time the health worker is in the area. Since people's health problems arise from their daily routines, every effort should be made to observe people engaged in daily activities. This can only happen when community members feel comfortable with the health care worker. For this to occur, the health care worker must spend time in the community and must be accepted by the community. Although this process of assimilation is time-consuming, it is the best method for observing candid community activity.

Studies which rely solely on brief community surveys risk collecting inaccurate information. R.S. Arole (1977) [4] found that when a professional survey team studied the incidence of abortion in Maharashtra, India, they grossly underestimated the incidence because women would not report such a delicate matter to unfamiliar outsiders. The women accurately reported a history of abortion to a local health worker who was well known in the community.

By combining the techniques of social anthropology with classical survey-based studies, the accuracy of information obtained is enhanced. Time spent living with community members adds depth and validity to the numbers collected during surveys. A balance must be achieved between the time needed for assimilation and the need to produce useful information promptly.

References

1. WHO, (1988). *Education for Health*:180-185.
2. WHO, (1979). Community Involvement in Primary Health Care. Report of a Workshop held in Kintampo, Ghana, 3-14 July 1978.
3. Williams C. D., Baumslag N., Jelliffe D. B., (1985). *Mother and Child Health: Delivering the Services*, Second Edition, Oxford Medical Publications:185.
4. Arole, R. S., (1977). Community Action - Family Health Programmes Delivering an Integrated Package. Illustrative Case Study: India, a paper for the IUNS Working Conference held at the National Institute of Nutrition, Hyderabad; 17-21 Oct.

Chapter 3

Basic demographics

The demographic composition of a community offers an excellent starting point for assessment. Such population factors as size, age structure, density, fertility and mortality may suggest health problems. Available services and resources should also be noted. The information obtained can assist the health care worker in recognizing high-risk groups and can suggest common health problems. It also better defines the population and outlines the amount of resources necessary and available for interventions.

Information about the study population can be gathered from published reports. These reports often include the size and density of the population, the male-to-female ratio, the age composition, the literacy rate, the number of schools, the number of clinics, the fertility rate, the birth rate, the death rate, the average income and the main industry. All of these factors can impinge upon health. Health care workers should use published reports only as a rough guide because national statistics may not apply to local communities.

Upon arrival at the project site, the health care worker should observe the demographic makeup of the population. For small villages, the inhabitants may come out to meet a guest. This is an excellent opportunity to assess the approximate size and age structure of the community. The age distribution in LDCs is skewed toward younger ages because many children do not live into adulthood (Figure 3.1). Even a lack of people can be telling. If debilitated people are all that remain in the town, it may be that most able-bodied people are working or farming elsewhere.

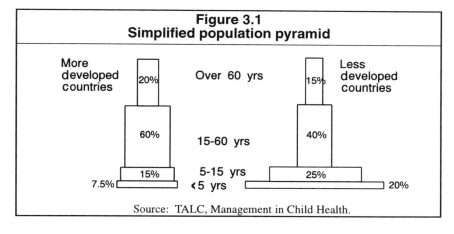

**Figure 3.1
Simplified population pyramid**

More developed countries: 20% Over 60 yrs, 60% 15-60 yrs, 15% 5-15 yrs, 7.5% <5 yrs

Less developed countries: 15% Over 60 yrs, 40% 15-60 yrs, 25% 5-15 yrs, 20% <5 yrs

Source: TALC, Management in Child Health.

Population density

An estimate of a community's population density is easily obtained and provides useful health-related information. The specific risks and benefits of high- and low-density areas vary. In general, people in high-density areas like cities have a longer life expectancy than do their rural counterparts. One reason for this is that city dwellers have better access to services such as medical facilities, clean water, sanitation and schools (Figure 3.2). Particularly important for pregnant women, transportation time from home to hospital is much shorter for urban inhabitants. Since a significant number of women die from easily treatable pregnancy-related complications, short transport times to health care decrease mortality.

High population density is one reason for better access to services in cities. It is more cost-effective to build a school in an urban area than in a rural area. One school in a city can educate thousands of people that live in close proximity to the school. In a rural area a number of schools must exist to educate the same number of people. The rural schools often require more resources and make monitoring intervention activities difficult. Other reasons for better service availability in cities include greater monetary resources, government officials directing service delivery to meet their needs first, and donor countries' preference for highly visible projects.

High-density areas are not without problems. Air pollution, road accidents, and violent crimes are more common in cities. Communicable disease transmission for such illnesses as measles, helminthiasis and tuberculosis is accentuated when people live in close proximity [1-3]. Because of rural-to-urban migration, many cities contain numerous unplanned slums where service delivery is nonexistent. Slum inhabitants receive little benefit from the increased population density, and risk increased disease transmission. A. C. Marques (1979) suggests that disease prevalence is increased in city slums due to inadequate services like water and sewage [4]. This results in epidemics of malaria and leishmaniasis.

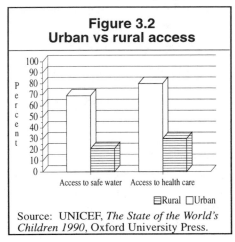

Figure 3.2
Urban vs rural access

Source: UNICEF, *The State of the World's Children 1990*, Oxford University Press.

Low population density can decrease interpersonal disease transmission, but the lack of services may offset any benefit. Rural communities are often composed of close-knit groups of people who maintain intimate contact with each other, but infrequently visit nearby communities. This suggests that transmission of certain communicable diseases is intense within a community, but transmission from village to village may be less common. Certain diseases may therefore display focal patterns of occurrence.

Faecal-oral disease transmission is an example of where the benefits of low population density are offset by the lack of services. A low population density means less garbage and excrement must be disposed of, but the services do not exist to meet the limited need. The result is cross-contamination from inadequately-handled waste products to unprotected water sources. Even in low-density areas faecal-oral disease transmission is intense.

Inhabitants of less populated areas generally grow the food they need while city dwellers must rely on local markets. This can insulate rural people from changes in international food prices. If the price of the staple food rises on the world market, the cost of feeding an urban family may rise beyond what the family can pay. Another positive aspect of low population density is that food production can be increased by improved farming methods. Therefore the rural farmer is insulated from world food prices and has the potential to increase the available food. A major concern for farmers is their dependence on environmental factors such as weather and pests. This results in significant seasonal variability in food production.

Many health problems are a result of population density. Estimating population density can guide the health care worker to common health problems. With the continual movement of populations from low-density rural areas to high-density urban areas, the problems of the urban slums will worsen.

Fertility rate and family composition

The fertility rate of women in low-income countries is high, resulting in large family size (Figure 3.3). This is most obvious in rural areas where large families are the norm. For the family, in particular the mother, a large number of children is significant. The more children a woman bears and the shorter the birth interval, the more likely she is to experience the

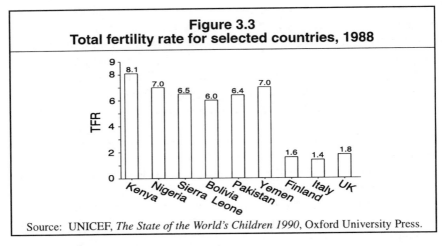

Figure 3.3
Total fertility rate for selected countries, 1988

Source: UNICEF, *The State of the World's Children 1990*, Oxford University Press.

maternal depletion syndrome and to die in childbirth (see box page 17). Short birth intervals also correlate with an increase in infant mortality (Figure 3.4). For families with similar economic status, the larger the family size, the more likely malnutrition will exist in the family. This is especially true for the child who is swiftly displaced from the breast due to a subsequent pregnancy. The translation of kwashiorkor is displaced from the breast.

The health care worker should take note of family size and the number of children each woman bore. A high fertility rate affects not only the family but also the entire nation. With a high fertility rate, some countries double their population every 20 to 30 years. Current problems will worsen as a growing number of people try to access an unchanging amount of resources. For example, for India to maintain its current level of education, it must build and operate 127 000 new schools each year. This is a result of 13 million children being added to India's population each year [6].

Figure 3.4
Relationship between birth interval and infant mortality

Spacing between births	Deaths before age one year, per 1000 live births
Less than 2 years	185
2 - 4 years	89
Over 4 years	58

Source: S. Rutstein, (1982). *World Fertility Survey Technical Bulletin: 2001*.

The age at which women begin having children and the total number of children they bear are two indicators of the status of women in their society. Early childbearing with short intervals between births suggests a low status for women. Their main worth, as seen by the community, is as reproductive machines. This trend has far-reaching implications for both women and the entire community. In general, the woman is the main caregiver and nurturer of the family. She is also a significant contributor to the income of the family. If the woman is sick or has died in childbirth, the children and the community will suffer.

Most traditional societies are based on the extended family structure with three or more generations living under one roof. This structure has many benefits including emotional support, guidance with such difficult tasks as breastfeeding and weaning practises, help with child support and supervision, and division of labor. With the urbanization trend, the extended family structure is disintegrating. Many young urban mothers feel isolated with no support for themselves or for their children. The health care worker should be aware of the family structure and any recent changes in that structure. Dwindling family support and city-based advertising encourages young mothers to see bottle-feeding as a viable option. Unfortunately, many of the urban poor lack the financial and educational resources necessary to bottle-feed adequately. This can be disastrous for the newborn's nutritional status.

Maternal depletion syndrome

The maternal depletion syndrome often begins at birth. In many cultures a female child receives less food and less health care than does a male sibling. This increases the risk of stunting and ill health even at an early age. Girl children are expected to work very hard to help the family. With menarche, the adolescent girl has an increased energy drain while at the same time is expected to work harder. Some cultures also place dietary restrictions on menstruating females. Early marriage and pregnancy place further demands on the body of a young woman who is still growing. Food energy is directed to meeting the needs of the growing foetus and, after delivery, milk production, rather than to completing the adolescent's growth. Throughout pregnancy and shortly after delivery a woman is required to work in the fields, care for the family, collect water and firewood, and do the cooking and cleaning. Closely-spaced births prevent a woman's body from recovering. With each successive pregnancy, the woman has fewer bodily reserves. This results in anaemia, protein energy malnutrition, stunting, goitre and decreased work output. The final outcome of this vicious cycle is the death of the woman.

The urbanization trend has resulted in an increase in the number of single-parent households headed by women. Up to one third of all families are now dependent solely on the income of women [7]. Single women who head households have a difficult time providing and caring for their families. Research suggests that woman-headed households have a higher incidence of malnutrition and infant mortality [8]. In part this is due to the overwhelming amount of work that must be done by one person. In addition, societies place women at a significant disadvantage. Women are frequently excluded from owning land, have difficulty obtaining credit and are denied certain jobs.

The traditional family structure can also adversely affect health. Many traditional families sleep in a common bed. Communicable disease transmission is therefore accentuated. This country bed can offset the inherent decreased disease transmission present in areas of low population density.

In rural India, it is common for the husband's mother to control much of the family's activities [9]. Even if the wife is educated, she may be forced to use unsafe feeding practises because household decisions are made by the mother-in-law and not by the wife.

The ratio of men to women is another important demographic point to note. If women predominate, it may suggest that men moved to the cities to look for work, or that wars or employment accidents have resulted in high mortality rates for men. If men predominate, female infanticide may be practised. In one community in China, there were five male infants for every one female infant [10].

The ratio of men to women in the household can provide clues to the prevalence of sexually transmitted diseases. In male-dominated societies, polygamy is common. As the number of sexual partners increases, the number of people at risk of sexually transmitted diseases (STDs) increases. With the introduction of the Acquired Immuno-Deficiency Syndrome (AIDS) into a community, the risk of contracting human immunodeficiency virus (HIV) infection will be greater for people in promiscuous polygynous societies than for monogamous societies. The prevalence of infertility due to fallopian tube scarring can also be greater in promiscuous cultures. Infertility is such a large problem that in some African countries close to 30 percent of women are infertile [11]. Much of this infertility is attributed to prior infections with chlamydia and gonorrhoea [12].

Socioeconomic indicators

Other basic demographic information pertinent to health includes employment opportunities, alternative sources of income, economic status, school availability, health clinic accessibility and environmental hazards. Although there are exceptions, a general trend in developing countries is an improvement in health as the family's income and educational level increases (Figure 3.5) [13]. Locating factories, markets, schools and health facilities may be easy. Identifying barriers to employment, education and health care is more difficult. Unless these barriers are discovered, successful intervention is unlikely.

For a family to increase their income, job opportunities and local markets must exist. If unemployment in cities is high and major industries which employ large numbers of people do not exist, the potential for improving income is minimal. Unemployment rates of 50 percent are not unusual. For rural farmers to increase their income, they generally have to grow more produce than their current output. Unfortunately, lack of available markets, poor product price and inability to transport the product to market deter the farmer from increasing profits. The health care worker should note any significant local industries or markets and the potential for gainful employment.

**Figure 3.5
Relationship between family income and infant mortality rate**

Family income per person (rupees)	Deaths before one year
Less than 20	180
Up to 50	82
Up to 100	46
Up to 200	18

Source: S. Ghosh, et al, (1979). *Ind. J. Med. Res.*, 69:616-623.

The earnings of women are significant, but national surveys tend to overlook this important source of income [14]. Women often make more money by selling in the market or by performing menial tasks than do men who work in local factories (Figure 3.6). With increasing financial pressures, women are at times taking over male-dominated careers such as blacksmithing, carpentry, or construction work. Women, realizing the significant disadvantage they have in finding work, are in some instances banding together to pool their resources and begin small enterprises. Women must be included when estimating family income or when planning income-generating interventions.

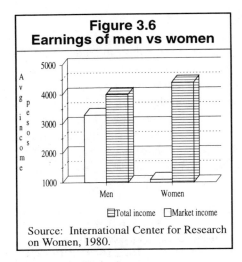

Figure 3.6
Earnings of men vs women

Source: International Center for Research on Women, 1980.

Just as women contribute to family income, so do children. In agrarian societies, children begin working on the farms at an early age. Farm-related accidents are common and children with limited experience may run significant risk of injury. In towns and cities, children are active sellers in the market. This can place children at considerable risk. An increasing number of children are killed in motor vehicle accidents. It is frightening to see young children dodging between speeding cars in busy streets just to sell a pack of gum to a stationary motorist. More deplorable is the use of child labour in sweat shops that manufacture clothing, rugs or other goods. Government regulations regarding child employment are commonly lax. Children often work long hours in unsafe conditions.

A family's health correlates with their economic status [15]. Except during the transition from a traditional subsistence economy to a cash economy, the nutrition of a family improves with higher economic status (Figure 3.7). A family's economic status can be estimated from what they own and how they live. The type of dwelling a family resides in is an easily identified indicator of family resources. A family that lives in a home constructed of imported materials is likely to have more resources than a family that lives in a home built of locally available materials. Personal belongings such as bicycles, cars, radios, televisions, animals and land can suggest the financial security of the family. Based on these factors, the health care worker can estimate the economic status of community members.

The education system is another demographic factor which health care workers should note. Are schools available, and if so, what percentage of the eligible population attends? Even when schools are available, the percentage of children attending school may be low. Barriers to attending school include the prohibitive cost of attendance, the great distance between home and school, the need for the child to work at home, the number and the quality of teachers. In some cultures, girls or certain castes are not allowed to attend schools. It is common for the literacy rate of male

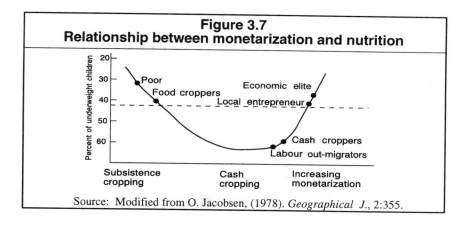

Figure 3.7
Relationship between monetarization and nutrition

Source: Modified from O. Jacobsen, (1978). *Geographical J.*, 2:355.

children to be much higher than that of female children [16]. This is unfortunate since improvements in a family's health are more closely linked to the educational level of the woman than of the man (Figure 3.8) [17].

Uncontrolled pollution of the environment with its subsequent health risks to the employee and the community is an issue. Major factories often use hazardous chemicals, but fail to provide protection for the employee. Occupational safeguards are not in place, and debilitating injuries to workers are common. When a worker is injured, the maimed worker is fired from the job with no benefits. Rural workers may be no safer from noxious chemicals than are their city counterparts. The health risks of fertilizers and pesticides may be unknown or protective equipment unavailable. These occupational hazards extend beyond the workplace. Community members are at risk from inadequately-disposed toxic pollutants.

Summary. Basic demographics provide an excellent opportunity for a health care worker to observe factors which affect health and are indicators of ill health. The health care worker can begin studying a population even before arrival in the community by viewing published statistics. Beginning with this search through the relevant literature, the health care worker can make simple observations of the community which will reveal

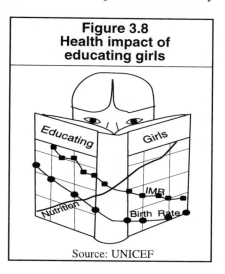

Figure 3.8
Health impact of educating girls

Source: UNICEF

problem areas. Next, the health care worker can either formulate possible solutions to the problems or begin a rigorous study of a problem highlighted during the initial survey.

References

1. Aaby P., et al, (1988). 'Measles Mortality: Further Community Studies on the Role of Overcrowding and Intensive Exposure', *Rev. Infect. Dis.*, 10:474-477.
2. Aaby P., (1988). 'Malnutrition and Overcrowding/Intensive Exposure in Severe Measles Infection: Review of Community Studies', *Rev. Infect. Dis.*, 10:478-491.
3. Chiwuzie J. C., (1986). 'Social Class and Susceptibility to Disease: A Study in the University of Benin Teaching Hospital, Benin City, Nigeria', *Hlth. Hyg.*, 7:76-79.
4. Marques A. C., (1979). (Internal Migration and Major Endemics), *Revista Brasileira de malariologia e doencas tropicais*, 31: 137-158. (in Portuguese)
5. Brown K. H., Black R. E., Becker S., (1982). 'Seasonal Changes in Nutrition Status and the Prevalence of Malnutrition in a Longitudinal Study of Young Children in Rural Bangladesh', *Am. J. Clin. Nutr.*, 36:303-313, August.
6. Bulletin UNESCO Regional Asia Office. 22:June 1981
7. Sivard R.L., (1985). Women: A World Survey. World Priorities, Washington, D.C.
8. Williams C. D., Baumslag N., Jelliffe D. B., (1985). *Mother and Child Health: Delivering the Services*, Second Edition, Oxford Medical Publications, p.60.
9. Williams C. D., et al, *Mother and Child Health*, p. 20.
10. Women of China (1983). *Why Female Infanticide Still Exists in China?* China Publications Centre, Bejing, China (May),1.
11. Belsey M. A., (1976). 'The Epidemiology of Infertility: A Review with Paticular Reference to Sub-Saharan Africa', *Bull. WHO*, 54:319-341.
12. Mabey D. C. W., Ogbaselassie J. N., Robertson J. N., et al, (1985). 'Tubal Infertility in the Gambia: Chlamydial and Gonococcal Serology in Women with Tubal Occlusion Compared with Pregnant Controls', *Bull. WHO*, 63(6):1107-1113.
13. Caldwell J. C., McDonald P., (1981). Influence of Maternal Education on Infant and Child Mortality - Levels and Causes, Liege, International Population Conference, Manila 1981, Vol. 2:79-96.
14. United Nations, (1978). Country Report on Women in North Africa: Libya, Morocco, Tunisia, African Training and Research Center for Women, United Nations Economic Commission for Africa, New York.
15. Nwosu A. B. C., (1983). 'The Human Environment and Helminth Infections: A Biomedical Study of Four Nigerian Villages', In: *Human Ecology and Infectious Diseases*, Eds: Croll NA and Cross JH, Academic press, New York, pp. 225-252.

16. Morley D., Lovel H., (1990). *My Name is Today*, MacMillan Publishers, p. 47; UNESCO. (1978) Estimates and Projections of Illiteracy. Document CSR-E-29. Paris: UNESCO
17. Morley D., Lovel H., (1990). *My Name is Today*, p.95.

Chapter 4

Water and sanitation

Water is a basic requirement of life that many of us take for granted. It is intimately associated with health. For people in low-income countries, water not only sustains life but also is a major cause of morbidity. Water is a medium for the transmission of such pathogens as bacteria, amoeba, parasites and viruses. Table 4.1 classifies water-related diseases into four groups.

In addition to the role of water in disease transmission, the inordinate amount of time and energy expended on water collection can adversely affect health. Given the importance water plays in the sustenance of life, the health care worker must assess the quality and availability of water in the community.

Water quality

Ground water from open streams and open wells can be a source of illness. Contamination of water occurs when people and animals use the stream for urinating, defecating and bathing purposes. The water from an open well is often obtained by lowering a bucket into the water. The bucket and the hands that touch it introduce infectious agents into the well water. An open well may also attract small animals and birds which can transmit pathogens. Communities that use open water sources often have seasonal variation in water-borne illnesses; the rainy seasons are generally worse [2]. Although results obtained from studies investigating the introduction

Table 4.1
Classification of water-related diseases

a) faecal-oral (water-borne or water-washed): diarrhoeal diseases, infectious hepatitis, etc.
b) water-washed only: scabies, conjunctivitis.
c) water-based: dracunculiasis, trachoma.
d) water-related, insect-vector-transmitted: malaria, onchocerciasis.

Source: Modified from Sharon Huttly, (1990). *Wrld. Hlth. Stats. Quart.* [1].

of closed well systems into a community have varied, it is generally believed that closed water systems are safer and probably reduce the risk of disease incidence [3].

A deep borehole, closed well system is an excellent source of water [4]. Unfortunately, it is expensive to install since a drilling rig must bore the hole, then a concrete foundation must be placed around the borehole, and a handpump must be attached to the cement in a watertight fashion. If the seal between the pump and the borehole is not watertight, contamination can occur. It is important for the health care worker to note if the well and pump are operational, and identify what mechanism is used to repair the pump when it fails. The most successful water projects are those that have community participation such as the formation of a pump committee which has responsibility for maintenance and repairs [5].

For larger communities a closed pipe system may be present. This is an excellent system when used correctly [6]. It involves having a large water supply available that is delivered by way of a closed pipe system to each neighbourhood or each home. One potential problem is the source of the water. If the water comes from a river or reservoir, but is not treated, the quality of the water is no better than that obtained from an open water source [4]. For large cities which have water treatment facilities, intermittent shortages of imported chemicals needed to purify the water may lead to tainted water. Sometimes poorly maintained pipes allow contaminants into the water supply [4]. With the continual expansion of unplanned urban slums, an increasing number of people lack access to safe water.

Water scarcity is becoming a problem in urban slums. Many people must buy their water from businessmen. The entrepreneur may provide a needed service, but the cost of the water can severely strain the finances of a family and result in the family obtaining less water than is actually needed for a healthy existence. Some poor families pay close to 30 percent of their total income for water [7]. However, there is no guarantee that the water is pure.

Most people who do not have water piped to their dwelling must store their water in a container. This water container may be a source of contamination of otherwise clean water. It is often overlooked as a source of disease transmission [8-12]. The studies by J. V. Pinfold (1990) [11,12] suggest that the majority of water contamination occurs during the storage process and that contamination at the source is minimal in comparison (Figure 4.1). Water containers should be intermittently emptied and washed. If possible they should be allowed to dry out completely in the sun. The use of a water container that has a spigot can also decrease bacterial water contamination.

J. V. Pinfold (1990) [11,12] also demonstrated that the method employed to wash dishes can result in increased bacterial exposure. In the study population, many people let their dirty dishes soak for hours in standing water.

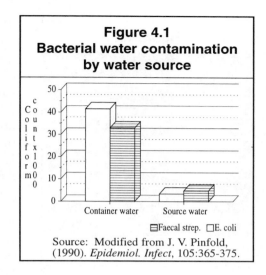

Figure 4.1
Bacterial water contamination by water source

Source: Modified from J. V. Pinfold, (1990). *Epidemiol. Infect*, 105:365-375.

This dishwater became grossly contaminated over time. People often completed dish-washing shortly before the next meal. As a result, meals were served on dishes still wet with contaminated water. With education, this practise of soaking dishes decreased.

Water quantity

When the quantity of water available to a household is limited, the risk of morbidity increases [13-15]. This is thought to be due to limited hygienic practises. It has been shown that proper hand-washing can reduce the incidence of diarrhoeal diseases by 20 percent. The two main barriers to hand-washing are ignorance regarding the need to wash hands and the limited availability of water. Proper hygiene education alone can reduce diarrhoeal incidence by 14 - 48 percent [16]. B. Stanton and J. Clemens (1987) [17] showed that a simple educational programme designed to improve personal hygiene decreased the incidence of childhood diarrhoea. Soap does not seem to be as important as the quantity of water used and the friction generated. Health workers should note if hand-washing is routinely practised.

Water shortage may be one reason for this limit on water quantity. More likely, too great an effort must be expended in obtaining the necessary quantities of water (Figure 4.2). A number of studies from Africa suggest that as the amount of time required to fetch water decreases, the quantity of water used increases. This relationship applies to situations where wa-

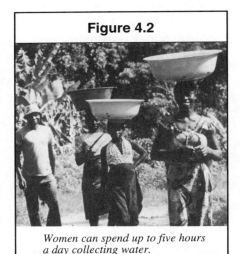

Figure 4.2

Women can spend up to five hours a day collecting water.

ter collection takes longer than 30 minutes. In addition, water consumption increases two- to three-fold when water is pumped directly to the house. Briscoe [18] summarized the results of a number of studies and found that women spend an average of two to five hours a day collecting water. Noting the length of time spent collecting water each day can enhance the health care worker's appreciation of the limitations on the use of water in the household. Interventions such as increasing handwashing must take this into account.

In addition to setting a limit on the quantity of water available, this inordinate expenditure of time and energy has significant repercussions on other aspects of life. A woman who must fetch water will spend less time meeting the needs of her children. This means a young child who requires four to five meals a day may be given food only once or twice a day [19]. She will also expend a great deal of her own energy obtaining water. A woman who walks for one hour to collect 10 litres of water expends close to 150 calories [20]. If the woman's caloric intake is limited, as is often the case, this high expenditure of energy may contribute to malnutrition.

Human waste disposal

In addition to proper hygiene, adequate disposal of human excreta is an essential step in breaking the faecal-oral cycle of disease transmission. In rural communities it is a common practise to defecate in the fields. Stool is a fertilizer, but it increases disease transmission. People may also defecate near a stream, thereby greatly increasing the range of contamination. Even when functioning latrines are available, people may choose to relieve themselves in their fields. There are many reasons for this habit. Some latrines are poorly designed, making the inside of the latrine inhospitable for even short periods of time. The latrine may not be in a convenient location. The farmer may feel his crops need the stool more than the latrine does. Where people urinate and defecate and the reasons behind their choices need to be assessed by the health care worker. In this way the health care risks and culturally acceptable solutions can be appreciated.

Children are particularly vulnerable to faecal-oral disease transmission. Their hygienic practises are inadequate to protect them from illness. Children tend to defecate and urinate in close proximity to their home. They also spend much of their time playing around the home. Consequently, this increases exposure to infectious materials. Given a child's important role as a disease vector and sufferer of faecal-oral transmission, it is especially important to note where children defecate and urinate.

Even city dwellers with flush toilets may contaminate the environment. A city's waste treatment plant may be unable to handle the volume of excreta delivered, or the plant may be temporarily out of operation. Heavy seasonal rains further increase the amount of excreta-containing water delivered to a treatment facility. This often exceeds the plant's capabilities to remove the contaminants. Human excreta will then be dumped directly into a nearby body of water. This water may be used for drinking and bathing purposes by other city dwellers.

Identifying where people defecate may be difficult. In many cultures, questioning about such delicate matters is inappropriate. Observation may be difficult because people go to great lengths to keep bowel habits private. The 'halo' effect is one potential problem that may arise when asking about bowel habits. For example, when a health worker questions a community member about the use of latrines, the community member may respond that the latrine is always used. However, this may not be true. The community member attempts to please the health care worker by providing an answer the community member thinks the health worker desires.

Disease transmission by water contact

Some water-borne diseases are transmitted by skin contact and do not require consumption. Schistosomiasis has a snail intermediate host that release cercaria that burrow into exposed skin. Therefore, the more time spent swimming, bathing or working in contaminated freshwater, the greater the risk of serious *Schistosoma* infections [21,22]. A protected water source such as a deep borehole well does not support *Schistosoma* transmission. Unfortunately, even in communities where a protected water supply exists, people will bathe or do laundry in an unprotected water source [23]. Because of such findings, all water sources need to be identified.

Health care workers can gain information regarding schistosomiasis prevalence either from published reports or regional health experts. If schistosomiasis is known to be present and people are involved in water-related activities, this parasitic infection can be a significant cause of morbidity. Although not specific, gross haematuria can suggest *Schistosoma* infection. Haematuria has been used as a screening tool for estimating the disease's prevalence (see Chapter 8, page 110).

Guinea worm (dracunculiasis) is another serious water-based parasitic infection. It is the only water-related infection that can be eradicated entirely by water supply improvements. If a person harbouring a female guinea worm exposes the infected extremity to cool water, the gravid female will release infective larvae. Ingestion of this larvae-containing water results in the infection of a new host. The unfortunate individual with dracunculiasis will be disabled for a number of weeks. Since the person most likely to be infected is the young adult who is the family provider, a prolonged disability can result in a significant decrease in family income and food [24-26]. When the mother is disabled by guinea worm infection, child care suffers [27]. Because guinea worm ulcers are obvious, health care workers can estimate disease prevalence by casual observation.

Water-related diseases

Other water-related infections include malaria and onchocerciasis. Malaria is transmitted by an *Anopheles* species mosquito which requires standing water for part of its life cycle. Onchocerciasis, which can cause blindness, requires transmission by the *Simulium* black fly (Figure 4.3). This fly prefers fast-flowing rivers. Areas surrounding rivers are often the most fertile farm areas, but their use has been severely limited by the presence of infected black flies [28].

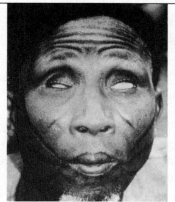

**Figure 4.3
Onchocercal blindness**

Source: MSD, Mectizan Product Monograph, 1988.

These water-related infections must be remembered both when assessing possible health risks as well as when contemplating health interventions. Many well-meaning agricultural projects have improved crop yield, but at the same time have increased the population's morbidity and mortality by creating habitat suitable for disease transmission. When moving from upland rice techniques to wetland rice methods, the potential exists for increasing the prevalence of malaria and schistosomiasis. With the building of Egypt's Aswan dam in the 1960s, the rate of schistosomiasis went from near 0 to 80 percent [29].

Summary. Clean water is essential for life. Recent research suggests that the quantity of clean water may be at least as important as the quality of the water. Personal hygiene and adequate sanitation are also requirements for health maintenance. In addition to water's role in faecal-oral transmission of disease, water-specific habitats may increase parasitic infections for community members. Because of the relationship between health and water, the health care worker must assess water-related issues in any general community survey. Interventions must be planned with the role of water in mind.

References

1. Huttly, Sharon R. A., (1990). 'The Impact of Inadequate Sanitary Conditions on Health in Developing Countries'. *Wrld. Hlth. Stats. Quart.*, 43:118-126.
2. Baltazar J., Briscoe J., Mesola V., et al, (1988). 'Can the case-control method be used to assess the impact of water supply and sanitation on diarrhea'? A study in the Philippines, *Bull. WHO*, 66(5):627-635.
3. Esrey S. A., Feachem R. G., Hughes J. M., (1985). 'Interventions for the Control of Diarrheal Diseases Among Young Children; Improving Water Supplies and Excreta-Disposal Facilities', *Bull. WHO*, 63(4):757-772.
4. Moe C. L., Sobsey M. D., Samsa G. P., Mesolo V., (1991). 'Bacterial Indicators of Risk of Diarrheal Disease from Drinking Water in the Philippines', *Bull. WHO*, 69(3):305-317.
5. Elmendorf M., Isely R. B., (1983). Public and Private Roles of Women in Water Supply and Sanitation Programs. Hum. Organization 42:195-203. [from *Technology and Women's Health*, MacCormack]
6. Pinfold J. V., Horan N. J., Mara D. D., (1988). 'The Faecal Coliform Fingertip Count: A Potential Method for Evaluating the Effectiveness of Low Cost Water Supply and Sanitation Initiatives', *J. Trop. Med. Hyg.*, 91:67-70.
7. Zaroff B., Okun D. A., (1984). 'Water Vending in Developing Countries', *Aqua*, 5:289-295.
8. Baltazar J., et al, (1988). 'Can the Case-Control Method be Used to Assess the Impact of Water Supply and Sanitation on Diarrhea? A Study in the Philippines', *Bull. WHO*, 66(5):627-635.
9. Black R. E., Lopez de Romana G., Brown K. H., et al, (1989). 'Incidence and Etiology of Infantile Diarrhea and Major Routes of

Transmission in Huascar, Peru', *Am. J. Epidem.*, 129:785-799.
10. Feachem R. G., Burns E., Cairncross S., et al, (1978). *Water, Health and Development: An Interdisciplinary Evaluation*, London: Tri-med:121.
11. Pinfold J. V., (1990). 'Faecal Contamination of Water and Fingertip-Rinses as a Method for Evaluating the Effect of Low-Cost Water Supply and Sanitation Activities on Faeco-Oral Disease Transmission. I. A Case Study in Rural North-East Thailand', *Epidemiol. Infect.*, 105:363-375.
12. Pinfold J. V., (1990). 'Faecal Contamination of Water and Fingertip-Rinses as a Method for Evaluating the Effect of Low-Cost Water Supply and Sanitation Activities on Faeco-Oral Disease Transmission. II. A Case Study in Rural North-East Thailand', *Epidemiol. Infect.*, 105:377-389.
13. Huttly S. R. A., (1990). 'The Impact of Inadequate Sanitary Conditions on Health in Developing Countries', *Wld. Hlth. Statist. Quart.* 43:118-126.
14. Esrey S. A., Habicht J. P., (1986). 'Epidemiological Evidence for Health Benefits from Improved Water and Sanitation in Developing Countries', *Epidemiol. Rev.*, 8:117-128.
15. Esrey S. A., Feachem R. G., Hughes J. M., (1985). 'Interventions for the Control of Diarrheal Disease Among Young Children: Improving Water Supplies and Excreta Disposal Facilities', *Bull. WHO*, 63:757-772.
16. Feachem R. G., (1984). 'Intervention for the control of Diarrheal Diseases in Young Children: promotion of personal and domestic hygiene', *Bull. WHO*, 62:467-476
17. Stanton B., Clemens J., (1987). 'An Educational Intervention for Altering Water-Sanitation Behaviors to Reduce Childhood Diarrhea in Urban Bangladesh: II A Randomized Trial to Assess the Impact of the Intervention on Hygienic Behaviors and Diarrhea Rates', *Am. J. Epidemiol.*, 125:292-301.
18. Briscoe J., (1984). 'Water and Health: selective primary health care revisited', *Am. J. Pub. Health*, 74:1009-1013.
19. Popkin B. M., Solon F. S., (1976). 'Income, Time, the Working Mother and Child Nutrition', *Environ. Child Health*, 8:156-166.
20. FAO/WHO (1973) Energy and Protein Requirements, WHO Tech Rep. Series, No. 522, WHO, Geneva.
21. Barreto M. L., (1991). 'Geographical and Socioeconomic Factors Relating to the Distribution of Schistosoma mansoni infection in an Urban Area of North-East Brazil', *Bull. WHO*, 69(1):93-102.
22. Kloos H., Higashi G., Schinski V. D., et al, (1990). 'Water Contact and Schistosoma haematobium Infection: A Case Study from an Upper Egyptian Village', *Int. J. Epidem.*, 19(3):749-758, Sep.
23. el Kholy H., Arap Siongok T. K., Koech D., et al, (1989). 'Effects of Borehole Wells on Water Utilization in Schistosoma haematobium Endemic Communities in Coast Province, Kenya', *Am. J. Trop. Med. Hyg.*, 41(2):212-219, Aug.
24. Belcher D. W., Wurapa F. K., Ward W. B., Lourie I. M., (1975). 'Guinea Worm in Southern Ghana: Its Epidemiology and Impact on Agricultural Productivity', *Am. J. Trop. Med. Hyg.*, 24:243-249.

25. UNICEF, (1987). 'Guinea Worm Control as a Major Contributor to Self-Sufficiency in Rice Production in Nigeria', UNICEF, Lagos, December.
26. Nwosu A. B. C., Ifezulike E. O., Anya A., (1982). 'Endemic Dracontiasis in Anambra State of Nigeria: Geographical Distribution, Clinical Features, Epidemiology, and Socio-Economic Impact of the Disease', *Ann. Trop. Med. Parasit.*, 76:187-200.
27. Watts S. J., Brieger W. R., Yacoob M., (1989). 'Guinea Worm: An In-Depth Study of What Happens to Mothers, Families, and Communities', *Soc. Sci. Med.*, 29(9):1043-1049.
28. WHO, (1985). Ten Years of Onchocerciasis Control in West Africa: Review of the Work of the Onchocerciasis Control Programme in the Volta River Basin Area from 1974 to 1984, WHO Document No. OCP/GVA/85.1B, WHO, Geneva.
29. El Kholy, H. (1983). Impact of the Aswan Dam on Health and Nutrition in Egypt. Cornell term paper, unpublished.

Chapter 5

Food - preparation and nutrition

Undernutrition is a major contributor to ill health and premature death. Surprisingly, malnutrition may occur even when enough food is available. Social habits or cultural taboos can limit the amount and type of food eaten. Certain practises may actually increase the risk of infectious disease, thereby further increasing caloric demand. Nutrition-related issues are intimately tied to wellness. The health care worker must pay particular attention to nutrition during general community health surveys.

Maternal effects on child nutrition

A child's nutritional status actually begins before birth. An underweight mother has an increased chance of giving birth to a baby which is small for gestational age (Table 5.1) [1]. Maternal stunting is a sign of chronic undernutrition and can contribute to complications such as cephalopelvic disproportion. The health care worker should note the nutritional status of women of reproductive age. If a scale is available, the health care worker can weigh women who appear at risk of undernutrition. Pregnant women with a pre-pregnancy weight of less than 38kg are classified as high-risk pregnancies. In India, 24 percent of women of reproductive age are below 38kg [2].

In addition to maternal stunting, neonatal health is adversely affected by maternal anaemia [3]. Although research regarding the association between maternal and neonatal anaemia is conflicting [4,5], anaemic mothers

Table 5.1
Maternal characteristics associated with birth weight.
Values in percent prevalence

Maternal characteristics	Birth weight > 2500gm		Birth weight < 2500gm	
	Urban	Rural	Urban	Rural
Teenage pregnancy	11.0	28.4	16.9	38.4
Height < 140cm.	1.0	0.6	2.9	2.6
Weight < 40kg	9.9	18.9	28.8	38.6
Haemoglobin < 8g/dl	9.9	17.2	22.5	16.2

Source: National Institute of Nutrition, Hyderabad, India, 1980.

and their foetuses have an increased risk of death. The risk of giving birth to an intrauterine growth-retarded (IUGR) baby is greater in anaemic mothers than in non-anaemic mothers [6]. IUGR babies are known to have a greater risk of premature death than do their normal birthweight cohorts.

The reasons for the increased risk of maternal death due to anaemia are probably multifactorial. A mother with a low haemoglobin has fewer reserves in the event of a bleed from placenta previa or abruptio placenta. That means an anaemic mother who begins to bleed is in danger of dying more quickly than a woman with a normal haemoglobin. It has also been shown that people with iron-deficiency anaemia are less physically fit and less productive [7-11]. This may result in the anaemic mother being stunted and wasted because she is unable to cultivate enough food to maintain optimal growth. The impact of maternal anaemia is felt by the entire family. A mother who is unable to meet her own needs is ill-equipped to meet the needs of her children. Obviously, an anaemia-related maternal death has far-reaching repercussions on the nutritional well-being of the family.

Maternal iodine deficiency has a more direct effect on neonatal health than does maternal anaemia. Iodine deficiency remains a significant health problem (Figure 5.1) [12,13]. An iodine-deficient mother is likely to give birth to a child who is severely mentally retarded, dwarfed and possibly deaf. The risk of stillbirth and miscarriage is also greater from a hypothyroid mother [14]. Even in cases where overt cretinism does not occur, evidence suggests that brain development, IQ and hearing are adversely affected (Figure 5.2) [15]. By estimating the prevalence of maternal

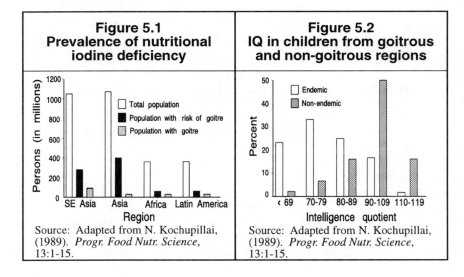

Figure 5.1
Prevalence of nutritional iodine deficiency

Source: Adapted from N. Kochupillai, (1989). *Progr. Food Nutr. Science*, 13:1-15.

Figure 5.2
IQ in children from goitrous and non-goitrous regions

Source: Adapted from N. Kochupillai, (1989). *Progr. Food Nutr. Science*, 13:1-15.

anaemia and goitre, the health care worker can assess the health risks to the newborn.

Child nutrition

Even before birth, a baby in a developing country faces many assaults on its nutritional wellbeing. These in-utero assaults can result in a low birthweight newborn. The newborn who weighs less than 2500gm is categorized as a low birthweight baby. This carries with it an increased risk of significant morbidity and mortality (Figure 5.3) [16]. Most low birthweight babies in the USA are pre-term babies, but more than 80 percent of low birthweight babies born in developing countries are believed to be full term. Maternal infections, malnutrition and genetic factors seem to play a major role in this discrepancy [17]. When food supplements were given to women with low pre-pregnancy weight and a low average caloric intake, the percentage of low birthweight babies decreased as did the neonatal mortality rate [18].

**Figure 5.3
Relationship between birth weight and infant mortality**

Birth weight(gms)	Deaths before one year
1500-2000	238
2000-2500	59
2500-3000	21
3000+	18

Source: S. Ghosh, 1978.

Following delivery, both underweight and normal weight babies face many obstacles to adequate nutrition. The health care worker must observe suckling and weaning practises to detect early causes of malnutrition.

Breast-feeding. The WHO recommends exclusive breast-feeding for the first four to six months of life (Figure 5.4). Then proper weaning foods may be introduced while breast-feeding is continued. Deviation from this has been shown to increase the health risks significantly for the baby (Figure 5.5) [19-21]. With urbanization and an increased exposure to Western culture, the rate of bottle-feeding has increased. In general, this is not an appropriate infant feeding method for a family with

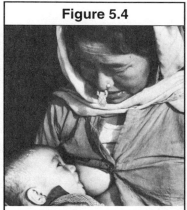

Figure 5.4

Breast-feeding is the best way for a mother in a developing country to feed her newborn baby. Source: UNICEF.

Figure 5.5

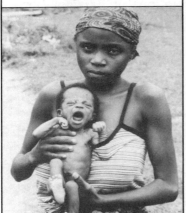

Bottle-feeding with dilute powdered milk formulas resulted in severe malnutrition in this six week- old infant.

limited resources. It may actually lead to ill health for the baby. Some mothers also introduce weaning foods well before the infant is four months old. Since weaning foods are often bacteriologically contaminated [22, 23], this practise increases the risk of infection and digestive problems [24-27]. M. G. M. Rowland et al (1985) [24] have demonstrated an association between early weaning and impaired growth in urban Gambian children.

Prolonged exclusive breast-feeding is almost as detrimental as weaning a child before four months of age. After approximately six months of age, an infant's nutritional needs grow beyond what breast milk alone can provide. If appropriate weaning foods are not introduced, the child may suffer nutritionally [28,29].

Weaning. The weaning period is a high-risk stage in a child's life. During this period, which occurs between six months and two years of life, malnutrition is a significant contributor to childhood morbidity and mortality. The weanling child is in a precarious stage. Breastmilk does not supply all the required nutrients, and the child's digestive system cannot process all types of food. Weaning needs to be a gradual process in which semi-liquid, easily digestible, nutritious foods are introduced and slowly advanced over time toward a more adult-like diet.

A number of less desirable practises occur with weaning that the health care worker should identify. Bulky, hard-to-digest, low-energy foods with limited nutritive value (e.g. cassava, white potato) are often introduced as the first weaning food. Young children cannot eat enough of these foods to supply all their caloric and nutritive needs. The food may not be adequately softened for the young child to digest easily. The diet may be advanced to a normal adult diet too rapidly. The child may be fed only twice a day even though the child's small stomach requires four to six small meals a day. The food that is given may have significant microbiological contamination which can lead to illness [22]. Desirable weaning foods, like fruits and vegetables, may be ignored in favour of the culture's staple such as rice, yams or corn. In some cultures, the staple crop attains an almost mythical importance in the minds of the community members. For people who enjoy highly spiced foods, the weaning food may be prepared with the same amount of spice as is used in the adult foods. All of these practises can lead to malnutrition in the weanling child.

The health care worker should identify the reasons behind the above-mentioned weaning trouble spots. If there is seasonal variation to food availability or family income, bulky low-density foods may be among the few foods available. Food may not be adequately softened or nutritious mixtures may not be prepared because of time constraints. For the woman who must work in the fields all day or away from home in an industry, the time required to prepare five or six fresh meals a day may not be available. Given the lack of adequate storage facilities for cooked foods (i.e. no refrigeration), the caregiver may need to cook five meals a day from scratch or serve food that was prepared earlier and run the risk of possible microbiological contamination. The woman may also need to cook the family meal to the exclusion of weanling food, because of a shortage of time, a limited number of pots and a limited quantity of fuel.

Food availability - family level

Even when nutritious foods are available at the family level, intra-family distribution problems may lead to inadequate calorie intake for certain members of the family. In many cultures there is a required eating order. The adult males eat first or get the best foods (usually animal protein). Women or possibly male children eat next. Finally, the young children, often female, are given what is left. This trickle-down effect may leave the last in the chain undernourished.

Another common eating scenario involves the use of a communal bowl. The entire family eats from one large bowl. This can place small children at a significant disadvantage, particularly if the quantity of food is limited. When no utensils are used and food must be gathered in the hand, the young child will be unable to eat enough food before it is eaten by the older members of the family. If utensils are used, the child may lack the digital dexterity necessary to transport food successfully from the bowl to its mouth before the communal food is eaten. Eating from a common bowl also increases the risk of transmitting infectious diseases from the contaminated hands of one family member to all other family members. One positive aspect that should not be minimized is the emotional bond which arises from a family eating together as a unit.

The family member who controls the purchase of foods may also determine the nutritional status of the family. The main caregiver and cook may understand how to prepare nutritious foods. However, if the person who decides what is eaten does not see the benefit of more nutritious foods, the undesirable practises may continue. When the man of the home is the main income-earner, a large percentage of the money earned may go to non-food items or expensive foods of low nutritive value (i.e. Western foods) [30]. The health care worker should identify both the cook and the person who controls the procurement of the foodstuffs. This will assist the health care worker in correctly targeting intervention strategies.

The cooking facility and cooking methods

Examining the cooking facility will provide information about other health risks. In homes where cooking is performed over an open fire, the kitchen is often separate from the sleeping quarters. In this way, exposure to cooking smoke is decreased. For people who spend a lifetime cooking over an open wood fire or for inhabitants of buildings where the cooking facility is attached to the sleeping quarters, the smoke may pose a significant health threat. Although research is scant, it is assumed that prolonged exposure to smoke may increase the risk of many pulmonary diseases including infectious, obstructive and cancerous types [31].

The method used to cook food and the fuel used can determine health risks. Open stoves or fires are inefficient. More fuel is needed to cook the same amount of food. They also increase exposure to harmful smoke. Closed cook-stoves are usually more efficient [32]. If the stovepipe is designed and functioning properly, exposure to smoke is decreased. A well-designed stove may also decrease the risk of burns (Figure 5.6).

Figure 5.6

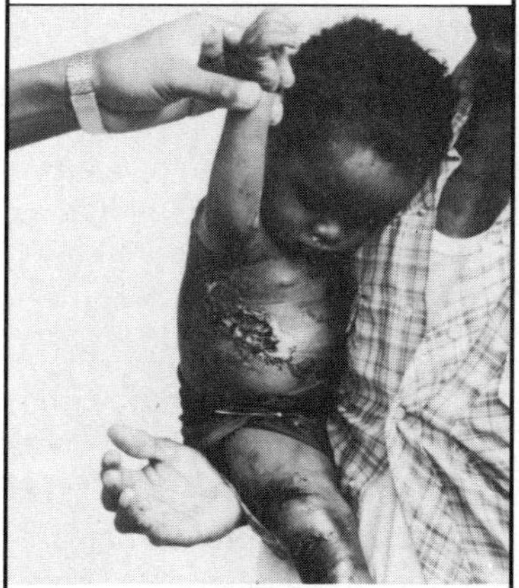

Child with multiple burns caused by boiling palm oil which was placed on a fire at ground level.

The introduction of fuel-efficient cook-stoves may have a significant impact on health in many communities. By increasing fuel efficiency, less wood or other fuel is required, thereby decreasing both deforestation and family expenditures on fuel. Deforestation and desertification are major concerns around the world as they have significantly decreased arable land. This in turn limits a community's potential food production.

Since fuelwood collection can take hours each day [33,34], a reduction in the need for fuelwood can result in a mother spending more time with her children (Figure 5.7). Well-directed time can result in improvements in the child's well-being. Carrying 10-30kg of wood for a number of miles significantly increases a woman's caloric expenditure [35,36]. Reducing the amount of work involved in collecting fuel for cooking can theoretically improve the nutrition of a woman if other factors are constant. This can lead to an improvement in the health of the woman.

Figure 5.7

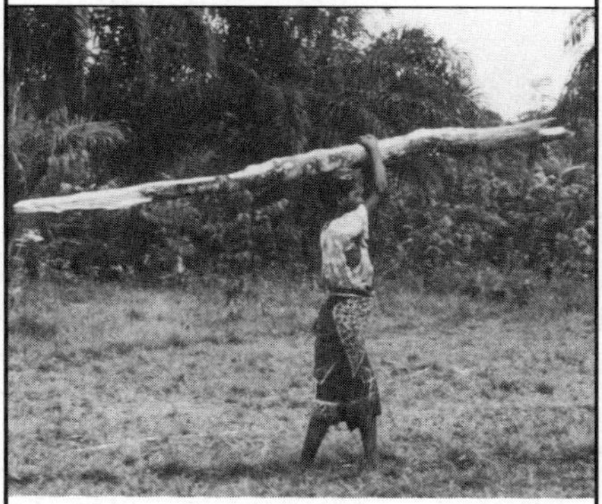

Gathering firewood takes precious time from a woman's day and requires significant energy expenditure.

When fuelwood is in short supply, women may alter their cooking habits to conserve fuel. This can result in inadequately-cooked foods, cooking less often, or briefly reheating leftovers [37]. Fuelwood shortage may result in a change in a family's diet. Since legumes often require prolonged cooking, removing them from the diet can save fuelwood, but the family's nutrition may suffer [38]. Fuelwood shortage may also lead to a change from cooking many-pot meals to one-pot meals [38]. In the final analysis Brouwer et al (1989) [40] felt that fuelwood shortage had a negative outcome on the nutritional status of families.

Cooking and storage of food affects health status. As mentioned above, the number of cooking utensils available affects how food is prepared. When the number of pots is limited, only one type of meal can be prepared. This limits the preparation of special weaning foods. It also limits the types of meals possible. Often one pot is used to cook the staple and a smaller pot is used to cook the topping. This may limit the amount of change a health care worker can introduce into the diet. Any change, such as the introduction of multimixes (Table 5.2), must be based upon the number of pots available.

Table 5.2
Examples of multimixes

Type of mix	Ingredients
2 - Mix	Staple + legume or Staple + animal product or Staple + vegetable
3 - Mix	Staple + legume + animal product or Staple + legume + vegetable or Staple + animal product + vegetable
4 - Mix	Staple + legume + animal product + vegetable

Note: Vegetable refers to a dark green leafy vegetable or an orange vegetable. Compact calories (e.g. oils, fats) should be added to all mixtures when available.

Source: D. B. Jelliffe and E. F. P. Jelliffe, *Dietary Management of Young Children with Acute Diarrhoea*, WHO and UNICEF, 1989.

Poor sanitary practises during food preparation can increase the faecal-oral transmission of disease. Proper hand-washing by the cook and the availability of a clean surface on which to prepare the food are important. Utensils must be kept clean. Animals and children, both of which may frequent the kitchen, are significant disease vectors [41]. Their handling of food and utensils during the cooking process should be limited.

Food storage is another factor. Without adequate refrigeration, food is often stored in the cooking pot. At some later time, the food is either eaten cold or is reheated. In tropical countries, the climate encourages bacterial growth on food stored in this manner. If the food is not properly reheated, the bacterial contamination may cause illness.

Storage of highly perishable foods such as fresh meat, fruits or vegetables poses a particular problem. When an animal is killed for consumption, it must either be eaten in one sitting or it must be stored in some way. If improperly stored, spoilage or microbiological contamination of the valuable food may result. Some cultures employ preservation techniques to extend the potability of foods. These methods include salting, smoking, drying and changing by controlled bacterial degradation (e.g. cheese and yogurt). In communities where such techniques are not known, an improvement in nutrition can be realized by their introduction.

Food selection

The selection of foods for consumption is a major determinant of a family's nutritional status. Dietary selection may be based more on cultural or religious beliefs than on sound nutritional principles. Many people in the Far East believe in the hot/cold theory. Many people in West Africa feel hot pepper is a panacea. Some cultures restrict pregnant women from consuming certain foods in the belief that it will harm the foetus [42,43]. In other instances, people may just eat what they are used to eating and exclude all other foodstuffs because of lack of familiarity. The health care worker should identify commonly eaten foods, readily available foods that are not eaten, the reasons behind people's food selections and ways of improving people's food choices.

As stated previously, a community's staple crop may take on an almost mythical property. Community members may eat the staple exclusively while ignoring other nutritious foods. Even during times of food shortage, people may bypass readily available alternative foods in an effort to obtain a limited amount of the staple [42]. In Liberia people believe they must consume at least one rice meal a day or they will be too weak to work. In the 1970s, Liberians staged a number of rice riots during a shortage of rice, even though other staples were available.

When people focus so narrowly on one food, they may inadvertently create malnutrition. One food cannot meet all of the basic nutritional requirements. Ideally, people will combine the staple with a number of other foods to create a well-balanced diet. The concept of multimixes as outlined by Jelliffe and others provides the health care worker with a framework for developing a nutritious diet [44]. Ideally, the staple will be combined with a vegetable oil, a legume, dark green leafy vegetables and when possible some form of animal protein.

In some communities the staple is grown during one season and a legume during another season. This can result in the staple being eaten at one time of year and the legume being eaten at another. If the two were combined into one meal, the protein available to community members would be increased.

The health care worker must remember that the classification of food versus non-food is a cultural one (Figure 5.8). What is considered food in one community may not be considered food in another. While Westerners may enjoy chicken eggs, people from other cultures may find that practise

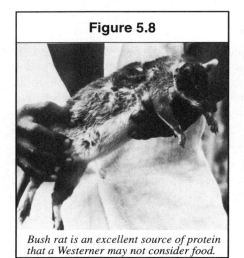

Figure 5.8

Bush rat is an excellent source of protein that a Westerner may not consider food.

abominable. The expatriate may have difficulty eating insects such as termite larvae, but it may be an accepted practise and an excellent source of protein in other cultures. A less dramatic example is when a Western health care worker tells a mother to find oranges to treat her child with scurvy. Oranges may not be locally available and the mother may spend hours walking and relatively large sums of money to obtain a few imported oranges. The health care worker should have suggested a more appropriate food such as pawpaw or mango which may be quite inexpensive and locally available.

To understand what foods are eaten and what foods are available, the health care worker needs to spend time in local markets and in members' homes. By approaching people in a friendly and inquisitive manner much can be learned about current nutritional practises. In time, methods of improving a community's nutritional status will be apparent.

Summary. Health is closely tied to nutritional status. Identifying the availability of food is an important first step in uncovering causes of malnutrition. The search must not stop there. Factors such as maternal nutrition, breast-feeding practises, culturally-based food habits, fuel source, and even the number of household pots all determine a person's nutritional wellbeing and, to an extent, their overall health. A general survey of a community is not complete without an assessment of these factors.

References

1. Oduntan et al, (1976). 'Correlates of Low Birth Weights in Two Nigerian Communities', *Trop. Geogr. Med.*:220-223.
2. National Nutrition Monitoring Bureau. Report for the year 1974-1979. Hyderabad: National Institute of Nutrition, 1980.
3. Brabin B. J., Ginny M., Sapau J., Galme K., Paino J., (1990). 'Consequences of maternal anaemia on outcome of pregnancy in a malaria ec area in Papua New Guinea', *Ann. Trop. Med. & Parasit.*, 84(1):11-24, Feb.

4. Iron Deficiency in Infancy and Childhood. Nutrition Foundation Report. International Nutritional Anemia Consultative Group, Washington, Dc, 1979.
5. Hercberg S., Galan P., Chauliac M., et al, (1987). 'Nutritional Anaemia in Pregnant Beninese Women: Consequences on the Haematological Profile of the Newborn', *Brit. J. Nutrit.*, 57:185-193.
6. Mahran M., Omran M., (1988). 'The Impact of Diagnostic Ultrasound on the Prediction of Intrauterine Growth Retardation in Developing Countries', *Int. J. Gynecol. Obstet.*, 26:375-378.
7. Basta S. S., Soekirman, Karyadi D., Scrimshaw N. S., (1979). 'Iron Deficiency Anemia and the Productivity of Adult Males in Indonesia', *Am. J. Clin. Nutr.*, 32:916-925.
8. Brooks R. M., Latham M. C., Crompton D. W., (1979). 'The Relationship of Nutrition and Health to Worker Productivity in Kenya', *East Afr. Med. J.*, 56:413-421.
9. Latham M. C., (1983). 'Dietary and Health Interventions to Improve Worker Productivity in Kenya', *Trop. Doct.*, 13:34-38.
10. Gardner G. W., Edgerton V. R., Senewiratne B., et al, (1977). 'Physical Work Capacity and Metabolic Stress in Subjects with Iron Deficiency Anemia', *Am. J. Clin. Nutr.*, 30:910-917.
11. Viteri F. E., Torun B., (1974). 'Anemia and Physical Work Capacity', *Clin. Haematol.*, 3:609-626.
12. Todd C. H., Laing R., Marangwanda C. S., Mushonga N., (1989). 'Iodine deficiency disorders in Zimbabwe. No change in prevalence of endemic goitre in Wedza District, as shown by school surveys carried out 18 years apart'. *Central Afr. J. Med.*, 35(1):304-6, Jan.
13. Ray S. K., Reddy D. E., Kaur P., Chaudhuri J. N., Tiwari I. C., (1989). 'An epidemiological study of goitre in two rural communities of Varanasi', *Journal Indian J. Pub. Health*, 33(1):9-14, Jan-Mar.
14. Hetzel B. S., Mano M. T., (1989). 'A review of experimental studies of iodine deficiency during fetal development', *J. Nutrition*, 119(2):145-51, Feb.
15. Grave G. D. (Ed), (1977). *Thyroid Hormones and Brain Development*, Raven Press, NY.
15a. Kochupillai N., (1989). 'The Impact of Iodine Deficiency on Human Resource Development', *Prog. Food Nutrit. Science*, 13:1-15.
16. Sterky G., Mellander L., eds, (1987). Birth Weight Distribution - an Indicator of Social Development, SAREC Report No. R:2, Stockholm.
17. Jelliffe, D. B. and Jelliffe, E. F. P., (1985). *Child Nutrition in Developing Countries: A Handbook for Fieldworkers*, Office of Nutrition, USAID, Washington, DC.
18. Lechtig A., et al, (1979). 'Effects of Maternal Nutrition on Infant Health: Implications for Actions', *J. Trop Peds*, 28, 273,.
19. West K. P., Chirambo M., Katz J., et al, (1986). 'Breast-Feeding, Weaning Patterns, and the Risk of Xerophthalmia in Southern Malawi', *Am. J. Clin. Nutr.*, 44:690-697.

20. De Freitas C. L., Romani S., Amigo H., (1986). 'Breast-Feeding and Malnutrition in Rural Areas of Northeast Brazil', *Pan Am. Hlth. Org.*, 20(2):139-146.
21. Holland B., (1987). 'Breast-feeding, Social Variables, and Infant Mortality: A Hazards Model Analysis of the Case of Malaysia', *Social Biology*, 34(1-2):78-93, Spring-Summer.
22. Rowland M. G. M., Barrell R. A. E., Whitehead R. G., (1978). 'The Weanling's Dilemma: Bacterial Contamination in Traditional Gambian Weaning Foods', *Lancet*, 1:136-138.
23. Black R. E., Brown K. H., Becker S., et al, (1982). 'Contamination of Weaning Foods and Transmission of Enterotoxigenic Escherichia coli Diarrhea in Children in Rural Bangladesh', *Trans. R. Soc. Trop. Med. Hyg.*, 76:259-264.
24. Rowland M. G. M., Goh S. G. J., Dunn D. T., Hayes R. J. (1985). 'Growth and Weaning in Urban Gambian Infants'. In Eeckels RE, Ransome-Kuti O, Kroonenberg CC, Eds. *Child Health in the Tropics*. Sixth Nutricia Cow and Gate Symposium. The Hague: Martinus Nijhoff Publishers: 9-18.
25. Watkinson M., (1981). 'Delayed Onset of Weanling Diarrhea Associated with High Breast Milk Intake'. *Trans R. Soc. Trop. Med. Hyg.* 75:432-5.
26. Barrell R. A. E., Rowland M. G. M., (1979). 'Infant Foods as a Potential Source of Diarrheal Illness in Rural West Africa'. *Trans R. Soc. Trop. Med. Hyg.* 73:85-90.
27. Barrell R. A. E., Rowland M. G. M., (1979). 'Infant foods as a Potential Source of Diarrheal Illness in Rural West Africa', *Trans R. Soc. Trop Med. Hyg.*, 73:85-90.
28. Waterlow J. C., Thomson A. M., (1979). 'Observations on the Adequacy of Breast-Feeding', *Lancet*, 1:238-241.
29. Jelliffe D. B., (1969). *Child Nutrition in Developing Countries, A Handbook for Fieldworkers*, USAID, Washington, DC.
30. Pandey M. R., et al, (1989). 'Indoor Air Pollution in Developing Countries and Acute Respiratory Infection in Children', *Lancet*, Feb 25: 427-428.
31. Stewart, Bill, et al, (1987). *Improved Wood, Waste, and Charcoal Burning Stoves: A Practitioner's Manual*, Intermediate Technology Publications.
32. Hoskins M. W., (1980). 'Community Forestry Depends on Women', *Unasylva*, 322:27-32.
33. Schenk-Sandbergen L., (1985). *Poor Rural Women and New Water and Fire Technology in Gujarat (India)*, Amsterdam: University of Amsterdam.
34. FAO/WHO, (1973). Energy and Protein Requirements, WHO Tech. Rep. Series, No. 522, WHO, Geneva.
35. Maloiy G. M. O., Heglong N. C., Prager L. M., et al, (1986). 'Energetic Costs of Carrying Loads: Have African Women Discovered an Economic Way?', *Nature*, 319:66-669.
36. Dasgupta S., Maiti A. K., (1986). The Rural Energy Crisis, Poverty and Women's Roles in Five Indian Villages, Technical Cooperation Report, Geneva: International Labour Office.

37. Eckholm E., Foley G., Barnard G., Timberlake L., (1984). 'Fuelwood: The Crisis That Won't Go Away', Earthscan Paper, London: International Institute for Environmental Development.
38. Alcantara E., (1986). 'The Domestic Energy Crisis, Women's Work and Family Welfare in Three Ecological Areas of Peru'. In: International Labour Office. *Energy and Rural Women's Work. Vol II.* Technical Cooperation Report. Geneva: International Labour Office.
39. Brouwer I. D., Nederveen L. M., den Hartog A. P., Vlasveld A. H. C., (1989). 'Nutritional Impacts of an Increasing Fuelwood Shortage in Rural Households in Developing Countries', *Prog. Food Nutrit. Science*, 13:349-361.
40. Black R. E., Lopez de Romana G., Brown K. H., et al, (1989). 'Incidence and Etiology of Infantile Diarrhea and Major Routes of Transmission in Huascar', Peru, *Am. J. Epidem.*, 129:785-799.
41. Vermury M., Levine H., (1978). Project on Beliefs and Practices That Effect Food Habits in Developing Countries, CARE, NY.
42. Williams C. D., Baumslag N., Jelliffe D. B., (1985). *Mother and Child Health: Delivering the Services*, Oxford University Press, Second Edition:21.
43. Ties Boerman J., Mati J. K. G., (1989). 'Identifying Maternal Mortality Through Networking: Results from Coastal Kenya', *Stud. Fam. Plan.*, 20(5):245-253, Sep/Oct.
44. Jelliffe D. B., Jelliffe E. F. P., (1989). *Dietary Management of Young Children with Acute Diarrhea*, WHO & UNICEF.

Chapter 6

Food - agriculture

There is a demographic shift taking place in developing countries as people move from rural to urban areas. However, at present 65 percent of people living in developing countries still reside in a rural setting [1]. Many of these rural inhabitants depend on subsistence agriculture for their food and income. Inadequate food production by these subsistence farmers is a contributing factor to malnutrition. As population size increases and people migrate from rural to urban areas, the need for increased agricultural productivity intensifies. This requires the remaining farmers to increase yield beyond subsistence needs.

Many Third World farms produce yields far below what is possible even when using improved labour-intensive techniques. Given the limited scope for expanding the current amount of land under cultivation [2], it is desirable to improve the yield from the land that is presently being farmed. In addition, much of a farmer's crop may be lost in harvesting and storage. This further diminishes an already small yield. The health care worker should identify possible bottlenecks in the agricultural system, and either offer solutions or direct the farmer to agencies that can help.

Food source and food availability

A community's sources of food need to be identified. In the rural setting, subsistence farming provides most of the food, although cash cropping is increasing. Families sell their main crop, and then buy their food from markets. In urban areas, local markets or stores provide the bulk of a family's food. In other settings, a family's main source of income may be pastoral-based. The well-being of their animals is thus dependent upon grazing land and water rights.

Many people obtain food from various sources; therefore, identifying all the food sources may require significant effort. The more numerous the food sources, the less likely the family is to suffer if one source is not available. Other potential sources of food that are currently not used by the community should be identified. These can include home gardening, animal rearing, fishing, hunting or even foraging. Once the main source of food is identified, closer inspection will reveal possible problems.

Seasonal Variation. In communities that depend heavily on one staple crop, seasonal variation in food availability can result in seasonal variation in the nutritional status of community members [3]. For communities with more than one growing season per year, the risk of seasonal food shortage decreases, but is not eliminated. Since most community members are painfully aware of seasonal food shortage, discussion with community members will guide health care workers in identifying difficult times of year. Solutions to this seasonal food shortage may lie in improving the yield of the staple crop, decreasing the loss of food in processing and storage, improving transportation methods, or introducing new types of food that will be available during staple crop shortage.

Land. In the rural setting land is often wealth. The most fortunate of farmers owns and works his or her own land. They pay little or nothing for their land and retain all profits or harvest. When land is scarce, poorer farmers must often rent land from richer land owners. Therefore, some of their yield must be used to pay for the land. The worst case is that of the indentured servant who must work a farm for the owner in an attempt to pay off a debt. In some cases the debt may have started a number of generations earlier. The indigent farmer's children will have to shoulder the responsibility of the debt as they reach adulthood. The debt often grows over time due to high interest rates and charges levied against the farmer for goods and other services. In this way the owner has, in effect, slaves who must do his bidding or face criminal persecution for failure to pay back money owed. This farmer and his family are at significant risk of undernutrition and ill health due to their lack of family resources (Figure 6.1) [4].

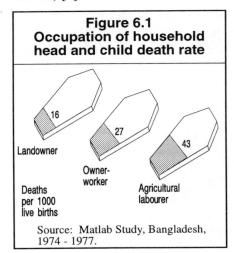

**Figure 6.1
Occupation of household head and child death rate**

Source: Matlab Study, Bangladesh, 1974 - 1977.

The land situation for single parent homes headed by women is even more bleak. Women may not be allowed to own land, and banks are hesitant to loan money to women. In this way, women are kept "in their place" with no hope for improvement in their situation. With the urban shift of population, men often leave women behind in the rural areas to care for the family. This has increased the number of single parent homes that are headed by women [5]. Until women are empowered, these women-headed households have little hope for improvement in their quality of life.

Factors limiting crop yield

While the main crops may differ between areas, labour-intensive farming is the norm. This is not expected to change in the foreseeable future [6]. In low-income areas, the purchase of expensive Western machinery is not possible. Furthermore, most farmers cannot afford the cost of expensive imported fossil fuels and lack the skill and spare parts to keep these large complex machines running. In addition, the social structure of small separate family plots of land is not conducive to large equipment use.

Many Western visitors to less developed countries see Western farming methods as the means to increase farm productivity. In many situations, this has actually decreased food production because the changes were not locally feasible [7-9]. Improvements in traditional farming methods need to be individualized and technologically appropriate. The health care worker can increase food availability by identifying and improving common agricultural factors that limit crop yield (Table 6.1).

1. Seed variety

In areas with minimal exposure to Western agencies, the seed used for the majority of crops will be traditional seed that has sustained agriculture for generations. Traditional seed usually produces a low yield, but is disease- and drought-resistant. This can have a moderating effect on crop yield. The variation in harvest quantity between a good and bad year may be small. Newly developed seed hybrids give better yields, but are often less resilient to environmental assaults. Therefore, if a high-yield seed were introduced into an area for which it was ill-suited, the yield may actually be less than that obtained with traditional seed. Because of this variability, great care must be taken when introducing new seed.

**Table 6.1
Common factors that limit crop yield**

Low-yielding seed
Inadequate irrigation
Inappropriate or nonexistent fertilizer use
Poor land management
Wasteful harvesting and processing techniques
Inadequate storage techniques

The higher-yielding seed generally requires a more favourable environment to achieve its 'superior' output. This means that irrigation techniques and fertilizer use must be optimized. Of note, even traditional seed will produce more if irrigation and fertilizer use are optimized. However, the increase in yield will be greater for a newer hybrid given the same level of improvement in other factors.

Local farmers and agricultural extension workers are the best source of information regarding seed type and farming methods used in the community. It is useful to note how familiar local farmers are with the agricultural worker and the quality of this relationship. Local farmers will sometimes mistrust a government-paid employee or may feel that a younger, book-smart person has little to offer. It is also helpful to discover what agricultural projects were attempted in the past and the outcome of each. If prior attempts at improving yield have met with failure, the local farmers will be reluctant to put much effort into yet another 'better method'.

Agricultural workers may be able to suggest newer, locally developed seed that has done well in regions that are similar to the target community. They may also suggest other techniques that can further improve yield. A number of agencies exist that have done extensive work in seed research and can offer solutions to identified problems (see Appendix, p. 135) [10].

The main cereal grains, rice, maize, millet, sorghum and wheat, have been improved significantly by plant researchers. Unfortunately, root crops, which many people in developing countries depend upon, have not been studied so extensively. Cassava, potato and yam research is minimal. The current potential for increasing yield of these important foodstuffs is quite limited [11]. This lack of research is in part due to the importance of the cereal grains to Northern countries which fund the research. Since the root crops are less important to wealthier nations, they remain neglected.

2. Irrigation
Crops require an adequate supply of water for proper growth. Most traditional farms depend upon seasonal rains to supply this moisture. A below-average rainfall causes a below average yield. Many farmers do not employ water control methods to utilize available water more efficiently. This fact, combined with worsening desertification and an expanding population, may spell disaster. Deforestation, a major contributor to desertification, leads to a loss of moisture-holding capacity of the soil. This results in a decrease in the amount of rain that falls. If crop yield is to increase to meet the needs of a growing population, some form of controlled crop irrigation must be implemented, and desertification must be halted.

Given the dependence on seasonal rains, the type of crop planted and the number of harvests per year will depend upon the number of rainy seasons. If only one rainy season occurs yearly, there will generally be only one harvest of the main crop. During the two to four months before harvest (the rainy planting season), food from the prior harvest is almost gone and undernutrition becomes more prevalent. This seasonal variation in undernutrition may highlight problems with food storage.

Potential water sources that can be controlled need to be identified. In areas with numerous streams, multiple options exist for controlled water use. Streams or parts of streams can be diverted to lower lying areas to provide all necessary water. Pumps may need to be installed on farms that are above available streams or that must rely on wells for their water. Some interesting pump designs are outlined in the literature including a foot-operated bamboo pump which is easily made from locally available materials [12]. Wind power or solar energy may also be harnessed to raise water to the required level. These naturally-powered methods are preferred to human-powered methods. Pumping water requires significant caloric expenditure. Most rural dwellers cannot afford this loss.

In hilly regions with water control problems, terracing, as is practised in South East Asia and China, may be an appropriate solution (Figure 6.2). Terracing involves putting step-like plateaus along a hillside. A water-retaining wall is built along the perimeter of each step. This wall holds water on the plateau that would otherwise run down the hill. By terracing a hillside, the entire hill becomes available for cultivation and has adequate water for optimal plant growth. Terracing does require an appropriate soil type that is not porous.

Attention should be paid to locally used methods of water control. As researchers have learned, the best and most culturally appropriate method of water control is often already available locally [13]. After failed attempts at small-scale water control in Somalia, researchers realized that the traditional methods known as gawan and caag were effective and culturally appropriate (Figures 6.3 and 6.4). They involve the use of earth bunds or ridges built in such a way as to follow specific contours of the land.

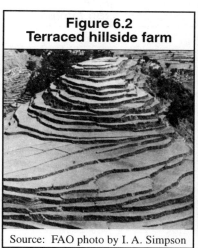

**Figure 6.2
Terraced hillside farm**

Source: FAO photo by I. A. Simpson

These bunds are constructed in various configurations to optimize water collection and retention. In this way, the small amount of rain that does fall is diverted and collected into growing areas.

When water is manipulated in some way, the potential health outcome of the intervention must be studied. If a stream is diverted, will this action affect people further downstream or will it harm other nearby farmers? If water is retained in standing pools, as is used for rice-growing, will the incidence of schistosomiasis and malaria increase? Without careful study, an irrigation project may increase crop yield, but worsen the general health of the population.

3. Fertilizer use

As the population continues to expand, the finite amount of arable land comes under intense agricultural pressure. Land that used to feed 10 people must now supply food for 15. Land that should lie fallow for three or four years must now be farmed every other year. The wealth of nutrients locked in the soil are being removed and not replaced. This nutrient-poor soil leads to crop yields that are inadequate to meet the needs of the people. Judicious fertilizer use can significantly improve yield.

Many farmers in developing countries use little or no fertilizer or use them incorrectly. Many reasons contribute to this practise, but ignorance may be the leading cause. Figure 6.5 shows the average use of inorganic fertilizer for selected countries [14].

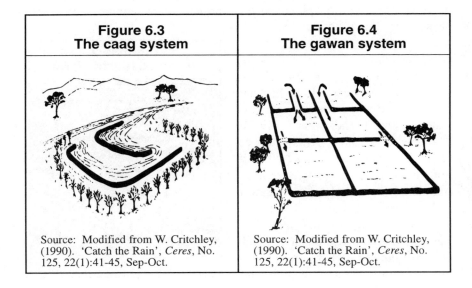

Figure 6.3 The caag system	Figure 6.4 The gawan system
Source: Modified from W. Critchley, (1990). 'Catch the Rain', *Ceres*, No. 125, 22(1):41-45, Sep-Oct.	Source: Modified from W. Critchley, (1990). 'Catch the Rain', *Ceres*, No. 125, 22(1):41-45, Sep-Oct.

In addition to ignorance, limited family resources, modes of transportation and availability of fertilizers contribute to underutilization. The greatest need for fertilizer use is in the rural agricultural regions. However, these regions have inadequate roads and limited transportation options. The rainy season is the time when fertilizer need is the greatest. It is also the time when roads become impassable. When vehicles are available, they are often expensive to run and difficult to maintain.

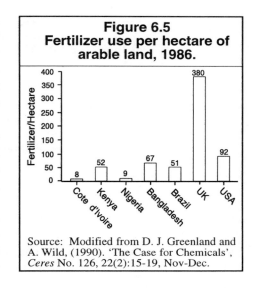

**Figure 6.5
Fertilizer use per hectare of arable land, 1986.**

Source: Modified from D. J. Greenland and A. Wild, (1990). 'The Case for Chemicals', *Ceres* No. 126, 22(2):15-19, Nov-Dec.

The type and availability of fertilizer depends upon local merchants who have little understanding of fertilizers. These merchants may buy the least expensive fertilizer, or the one that is easy to obtain. However, this may not be the best fertilizer. The three main plant nutrients that fertilizers supply are nitrogen, phosphorus, and potassium (N:P:K ratio). By monitoring the fertilizer consumption in Asian countries, it has been discovered that fertilizers too low in potassium are the most used type of fertilizer. After a few years of this fertilizer use, crop yield will be limited by a potassium deficiency. As NPK fertilizer use becomes widely accepted, micronutrient deficiencies such as zinc, copper, iron and manganese become more important [15].

As has been shown in Western countries, inappropriate use of man-made chemicals, like inorganic fertilizers, can lead to contamination of the environment [16-18]. Inadequate teaching of farmers in developing countries may result in environmental poisoning that adversely affects the farmer's health. The use of organic fertilizers is often overlooked by Western educators as a viable fertilizer method. Organic fertilizers have many advantages. One of the greatest of these is a decrease in the risk of environmental catastrophe (Table 6.2).

Some traditional farming methods rely on organic fertilizers. Increasing land and fuelwood demands have decreased traditional organic fertilizer use. The simplest organic fertilizing method involves leaving the plant

| Table 6.2
Advantages of organic fertilizers |
|---|
| Inexpensive
Locally available
Supply NPK
Supply micronutrients
Keep soil workable and aerated
Low risk of over-application
Low environmental risk |

stalk in the field after harvest. Because of the worsening fuel shortage, some farmers must harvest the stalk and use it for the cooking fire [19-21]. This is turn increases the nutrient drain on the soil. Animal dung is an excellent fertilizer, but it is being used with greater frequency as a fuel source (Figure 6.6) [22]. To combat this misdirected use of organic fertilizers, fast-growing leguminous trees and high-efficiency cook-stoves are gaining wider acceptance.

Leguminous plants make it possible for nitrogen-fixing bacteria to convert atmospheric nitrogen into a form that is available for plant use. One method of improving the nitrogen content of the soil involves planting fast-growing leguminous trees such as the *Leucaena* tree. The tree can be planted during a field's fallow period, and then can be harvested in a few years time for firewood. From planting until harvest, leguminous trees can make 40 to 70kg of nitrogen per hectare available for subsequent crops.

Figure 6.6

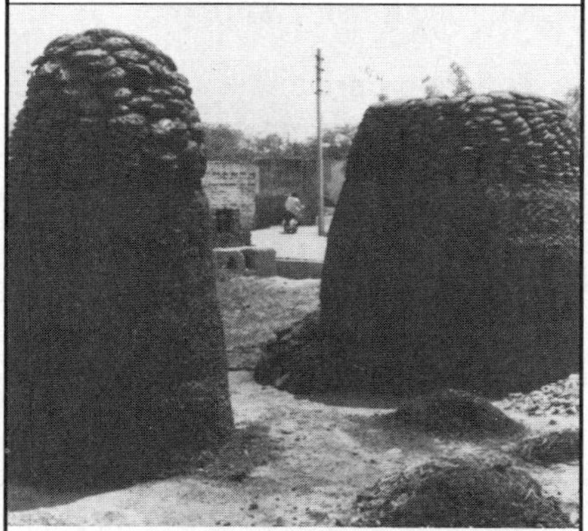

Cow dung is increasingly being used for fuel instead of fertilizer.
Source: FAO photo by I. de Borhegyi.

Since the trees supply firewood, the need for other fuel sources such as plant stalks and animal dung are decreased. This further decreases the nutrient drain on the soil.

Other nitrogen-fixing species are being used in a variety of cropping methods. One method uses intercropping. This involves planting a leguminous crop, such as cow peas or soy beans, between rows of the main cereal crop such as maize. Green manuring is another method of organic fertilization. A non-food leguminous crop is grown during a field's fallow year. The crop is then plowed under to increase the nitrogen content of the soil for the following year's main crop. Some thought has been given to using freshwater algae as an organic fertilizer. In the right situation, this may be appropriate.

Composting is an excellent method of increasing the nutrient content of soil. It is best used on a small area of land like a family's garden. Human waste can even be used if it is treated properly. Some improved latrine designs include a cooking chamber. Human waste is deposited in a latrine with a solar heater apparatus. This causes the chamber to get hot enough to kill all pathogens. After a few months the human stool is decomposed and sterile enough to be used as fertilizer. In China, human excrement is a valuable fertilizer. Stool is actually sold [23]. It must be remembered that improperly treated stool will greatly increase the chance of disease transmission.

The highest crop yield will be realized if both organic and inorganic fertilizers are used in concert [24]. When farmyard manure is used in combination with inorganic fertilizers, the yield can be increased by at least 20 percent beyond that obtained from using inorganic fertilizer alone. This dual fertilizer practise is a more realistic method for rural subsistence farmers because it decreases the need for imported fertilizer.

The health care worker needs to explore the use of fertilizers by local farmers. If fertilizers are used, are they used correctly and is there room for improvement? If fertilizers are not used, are there options available for the introduction of fertilizers? By observing farm activities, discussing fertilizer use with farmers, and by contacting agricultural extension workers, the health care worker can appreciate impediments to improved crop yields.

4. Land management

Land is a major resource for low-income countries. Unfortunately, the need to meet current economic difficulties has resulted in short-sighted exploitation of the land. This is true at both the governmental and personal level. Countries sell off their timber to foreign interests with no provision for replanting the destroyed forests [25]. This can be catastrophic to the land, as it results in soil erosion and desertification [26]. This severely limits land use in the future.

A Food and Agriculture Organization (FAO/UNEP) study in Africa suggests that 1.3 million hectares of forest are destroyed annually in Africa

(Figure 6.7) [27]. Foley (1986) [28] estimates that fuelwood reserves will be exhausted long before the world's oil fields are depleted. Given that up to 80 percent of a family's cooking and heating energy come from plant material, a fuelwood shortage would be catastrophic [29,30].

Even at the village level, land management may be a problem. The increased demand for firewood and the need to farm land until it is exhausted of all nutrients may leave the land unusable [31]. The health care worker should note if land is used in a renewable fashion.

Much can be learned about a government's use of land by examining its export statistics. If wood, iron, coal or precious metal etc. are contributors to the gross domestic product, abuses of the land may be occurring. The health care worker should inquire into the harvesting techniques used and the efforts made to replace removed resources. Viewing the harvesting activities may be enough to gain an understanding of the problem. Is replanting of forests occurring? Are coal and iron removed by strip mining? Is dredging used to collect precious metals? Are dangerous chemicals used in the processing of these metals? The poor of a country will be the first to suffer from inappropriate harvesting techniques. They are the ones who must make a living in the forest that is turning into desert, or must get their water from a river choked with silt or chemicals.

Change at the national level will be difficult. In the short term, the health care worker may have a greater impact at the village level. If fuelwood is scarce, finding alternative ways of cooking may decrease the pressure on the remaining trees. If excessive soil erosion is occurring, water management may decrease the damage and preserve the soil for later use. If farming techniques remove too many of the soil nutrients, judicious use of fertilizers may improve health. As the world's population expands, pressure for land will intensify. Without adequate management, the land will be unable to support a growing population.

Figure 6.7

Logging of tropical hardwoods destroys rainforests and endangers the long-term survival of nearby people.

5. Harvesting and storage
Even if a subsistence farmer uses a new high-yield seed, improved irrigation techniques and appropriate fertilizers, the food available for consumption may increase only slightly due to poor harvesting and

storage techniques. Grain, from the time of planting to the time of consumption, is being attacked by numerous pests. Birds, rodents, mammals, insects and microorganisms all diminish the food available for consumption.

Most subsistence farmers harvest their crop by slow labour-intensive methods. These methods may be inefficient and wasteful as some of the harvest is lost in the processing. When a farmer has a particularly bountiful harvest, the farmer may not possess the means to harvest the entire crop before it spoils. For the poorest subsistence farmer who cuts each stalk of rice by hand, the percentage of grains missed or lost will be small. If a farm animal is used, the percent wasted will increase, but the crop will be harvested faster. The health care worker should make a note of the harvesting methods used and the potential for waste.

Once a crop is harvested, it must be adequately and promptly prepared to avoid spoilage. For grain crops, the grain must be removed from the stalk, or threshed (Figure 6.8). It is then dehulled by removal of the outer coat (Figure 6.9). The grain may then be eaten, or it may need further processing such as milling. Inefficient threshing techniques can miss grain on the stalk or can damage the grain. Dehulling is generally time-consuming and grain is likely to be damaged or discarded in this process. Each time a crop is processed, some wastage will occur.

Adequate storage requires that the crop be prepared correctly. This involves reducing the moisture content of the crop. Even with adequate dry-

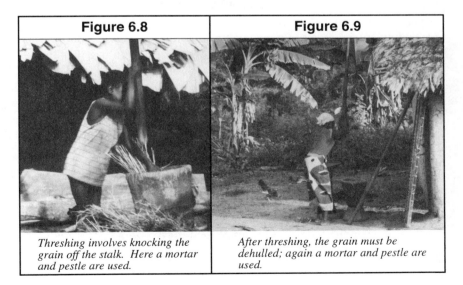

Figure 6.8	Figure 6.9
Threshing involves knocking the grain off the stalk. Here a mortar and pestle are used.	*After threshing, the grain must be dehulled; again a mortar and pestle are used.*

ing, an inadequate storage facility will lead to loss of food to rodents, insects and microorganisms. The storage techniques and facilities used should be observed. Agricultural extension workers may point out deficiencies in various aspects of each storage method and suggest simple improvements. Appropriate technology books exist which can guide the health care worker in designing improved storage facilities [32].

One simple method of increasing the amount of food available to a family is the preparation of a home garden. It is often overlooked in a community assessment and offers a very simple solution to the many nutrition-related problems. Even urban families may be able to have a garden. A 100 square foot plot of land (10 ft x 10 ft) can produce enough fruits and vegetables to improve the family's diet. Most fruits and vegetables provide required vitamins and minerals. As more is learned about the importance of adequate amounts of vitamin A for the maintenance of health, the need for a readily available source of vitamin A becomes apparent. This can be supplied by a home garden. Vegetables can even be planted along the edges of farms or in other unused pieces of land.

Summary. The majority of the world's population continues to live in rural areas where agriculture remains the primary source of food. Subsistence farming is the most common agricultural production method. For farmers to meet the needs of a growing population, improved methods of food production must be developed. By noting seed type, irrigation techniques, fertilizer use, land management, harvesting techniques and storage methods the health care worker will likely discover shortcomings of the current farming system. Once these are identified, viable solutions can be tried in cooperation with local farmers.

References

1. United Nations Fund for Population Activities. 1985 Report. p. 31.
2. Global 2000 report, U.S. Government, from Science, July 22 1983.
3. Brown K. H., Black R. E., Becker S., (1982). 'Seasonal Changes in Nutrition Status and the Prevalence of Malnutrition in a Longitudinal Study of Young Children in Rural Bangladesh', *Am. J. Clin. Nutr.*, 36:303-313, August.
4. De Freitas C. L., Romani S., Amigo H., (1986). 'Breast-Feeding and Malnutrition in Rural Areas of Northeast Brazil', *Pan Am. Hlth. Org.*, 20(2):139-146.

5. Williams C. D., Baumslag N., Jelliffe D. B.,(1985). *Mother and Child Health: Delivering the Services*, Oxford University Press, Second Edition:60.
6. Van Wambeke A. R., (1984). 'Land Resources and World Food Issues', *World Food Issues*, Cornell University.
7. Wharton C. R., (1969). 'The Green Revolution: Cornucopia or pandora's box?', *Foreign Affairs*, 47:464-476.
8. Pinstrup-Anderson P., (1981). Nutritional Consequences of Agricultural Projects: Conceptual Relationships and Assessment Approaches. World Bank Staff Working Paper No. 456. Washington, DC.
9. Pinstrup-Anderson P. and Hazel P. B. R., (1987). 'The Impact of the Green Revolution and Prospects for the Future'. In J.P. Gittinger, et al, Eds. *Food Policy*. Johns Hopkins Univ. Press, Baltimore MD: 106-118.
10. Pinstrup-Andersen P., Kennedy E., (1990). 'The Effects of Expanded Cash Crop Production on Income and Nutrition', *World Food Issues*, Cornell University, Vol 2:64-70.
11. Brun T. A., et al, (1990). 'Evaluation of the Impact of Agricultural Projects on Food, Nutrition, and Health', *World Food Issues*, Cornell University: 94-104.
12. tapak-tapak pump, IRRI, P.O. Box 933, Manilla, Philippines
13. Critchley, W. (1990). 'Catch the Rain', *Ceres* 125, Vol. 22, No.1: 41-45, Sep-Oct.
14. Greenland D. J. and Wild A., (1990). 'The Case for Chemicals', *Ceres* 126 Vol22 No2:18, Nov-Dec.
15. Tandon H. L. S., (1990). 'Where Rice Devours the Land', *Ceres* 126 Vol 22 No 2:25-29, Nov-Dec.
16. Ley D. H., (1986). 'Nitrite Poisoning in Herring Gulls (*Larus argentatus*) and Ring-Billed Gulls (*Larus delawarensis*)', *J. Wildlife Diseases*, 22(3):381-384, Jul.
17. Hutton M., (1983). 'Sources of Cadmium in the Environment', *Ecotox. Environ. Safety*, 7(1):9-24, Feb.
18. Tjell J. C., Christensen T. H., Bro-Rasmussen F., (1983). 'Cadmium in Soil and Terrestrial Biota, with Emphasis on the Danish Situation', *Ecotox. Environ. Safety*, 7(1):122-140, Feb.
19. Hoskins M. W., (1981). 'Community Forestry Depends on Women', *Unasylva*, 322:27-32.
20. Ki-Zerbo J., (1981). 'Women and the Energy Crisis in the Sahel', *Unasylva*, 33:5-10.
21. FAO, (1983). Rural Women, Forest Outputs and Forestry Projects, Discussion Draft. Rome: Food and Agriculture Organization.
22. Eckholm E., Foley G., Barnard G., Timberlake L., (1984). Fuelwood: The Crisis That Won't Go Away, Earthscan Paper, London: International Institute for Environmental Development.
23. Winblad U., Kilama W., (1985). *Sanitation Without Water*, Macmillan Education.
24. Braun A., (1990). 'Sustaining the Soil', *Ceres* 126, Vol 22 No2: 10-15, Nov-Dec.
25. Mercado, Juan, (1990). 'A Wasted Heritage', *Ceres* 126, Vol 22:42-46, Nov-Dec.

26. Cecelski E., (1987). Linking Energy with Survival. A Guide to Energy, Environment and Rural Women's Work, Geneva: International Labour Office.
27. Timberlake L., (1985). Africa in Crisis: The Causes the Cures of Environmental Bankruptcy, Washington, DC.
28. Foley G., (1986). Fuelwood: The Energy Crisis of the Poor, *The Courier*, 95:66-69.
29. Anderson D., Fishwick R., (1984). Fuelwood Consumption and Deforestation in African Countries, World Bank Staff Working Papers 704, Washington, DC: World Bank.
30. Brouwer I. D., Nederveen L. M., den Hartog A. P., Vlasveld A. H. C., (1989). 'Nutritional Impacts of an Increasing Fuelwood Shortage in Rural Households in Developing Countrie's, *Prog. Food Nutrit. Science*, 13:349-361.
31. Chavangi N. A., Engelhard R. J., Jones V., (1984). Culture as the Basis for Implementing Self-Sustaining Woodfuel Development Programmes, Nairobi: the Beijer Institute.
32. Small Farm Grain Storage 3: Storage Methods, Action/Peace Corps/VITA, 1978.

Chapter 7

Identification of community resources

Problems identified during a community assessment can only be addressed if the resources exist to implement interventions. During the identification of community problems, the health worker should note all available and potential resources. With this information, effective use of available resources can occur.

People

People are the most valuable resource in any community. Without their involvement, input and enthusiasm, intervention is not possible. There will be those who embrace change and those who strive to maintain the status quo. It is the health care worker's job to identify and encourage the liberal thinkers and minimize the negative effects of the conservatives. If entire communities do not want change, it is best to move on to more fertile ground. If interventions bring improvement to neighbouring villages, the conservatives may, with time, allow change to enter into their lives.

1. Leaders
Elected leaders are in power because of the positive image they project to community members. Leaders are important members of the society, and their attitudes and actions can influence others. Community leaders should endorse interventions, and if possible, take an active role in the interventions. This may entail the leader's children being the first in the community to be immunized. In this way others are encouraged to bring their children and are reassured that the procedure is safe. If the leader's wife breast-feeds, others will see breast-feeding as a prestigious and acceptable way of feeding newborns.

2. Skilled workers
Identify people in the community with special skills. Since many interventions require the assembly of equipment or the construction of buildings, skilled craftspeople who are willing to help need to be identified. This may include metal workers, blacksmiths, carpenters, masons, plumbers, electricians and others. People with special skills should be en-

couraged to assist in the project. Care must be taken when craftspeople demand payment for their services. If one person is paid, then all craftspeople will demand payment. This may be impossible given a community's limited financial resources.

Use skilled workers who live in the project site and avoid bringing similarly skilled workers from outside. Ignoring local workers in favour of outside labour can result in the shunned worker taking an active role to halt the planned intervention. If outside workers must be used, every effort should be made to include the local craftsperson. The hope is that by using only community members, the community will take pride in their accomplishments while at the same time decreasing the monetary cost of the project. This will increase the likelihood of success and can encourage community members to maintain the intervention long after the current health worker is gone.

3. Literate people

Community members who can read and write are particularly valuable. Most health surveys require some method of recording data. Ideally, health survey responses will be obtained by community members who can read and write. A literate community health worker or traditional birth attendant has more freedom in communicating with health workers in distant referral centres than does their illiterate counterpart. Educated literate community members can play a role in education. It should be noted that reading skill is not the only criterion on which to base selection for a particular task. An enthusiastic illiterate person who is honest may be more desirable as a community health worker (CHW) than a dishonest, uninterested literate person.

4. Community members

Able-bodied community members who support interventions are essential for the success of projects. They are the ones who have the most to gain from improvements, and they constitute the majority of the population. Health care workers from outside the community cannot do all the work. The majority of the effort must come from community members.

5. Traditional healers

Western-trained health care professionals often interact with traditional healers in an adversarial manner. This is unfortunate. Traditional healers play an important role in their society and meet a certain need. Their remedies may be more efficacious than Westerners are willing to admit. Traditional healers should be sought out, identified and encouraged to take part in health interventions (Figure 7.1). Some healers want to improve their skills and see Western medicine as a means to that end. Westerners can learn about traditional disease beliefs, culturally appropriate interpersonal interaction techniques, and viable treatment alternatives. The inclusion of traditional healers can enrich health intervention projects.

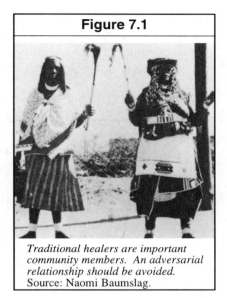

Figure 7.1

Traditional healers are important community members. An adversarial relationship should be avoided.
Source: Naomi Baumslag.

Raw materials

Raw materials are necessary for most interventions. Buildings, storage facilities, latrines, roads, cook-stoves, etc. all require raw materials for construction. Indigenous people have used locally available materials for centuries because they are easily obtained and are functional. The health care worker must identify commonly used materials (Table 7.1), and note their cost, availability, and range of applicability. Consideration must also be given to viable alternatives, both domestic and imported.

1. Building materials

People adapt available raw materials to their purpose. Where wood is available and termites do not exist, it is the main building material. Desert

Table 7.1
Examples of local building materials

Mud	Thatch
Termite dirt	Cement
Adobe bricks	Ceramics
Wood - timber and processed	Garbage
Bamboo	Plant stalks
Metal	

dwellers use available clay to construct adobe buildings. Affluent community members may use cement blocks for construction because of improved durability. The time-proven wisdom of building material selection must be heeded, and substitution with alternative materials should only occur after careful consideration.

Learn where the building materials are obtained. Note how much work goes into the collection and preparation of these materials. Learn the average life expectancy of each material. Where alternatives exist, study the pros and cons of each choice.

In south-east Liberia, roofing material is of two types (Figure 7.2). The traditional method of roofing involves collecting plant leaves (thatch) from the surrounding jungle and tying these to the wood poles that form the supports of the roof. It makes a waterproof roof that helps keep the inside of the house cool, and costs nothing to build. One drawback to thatch roofs is the amount of work involved in collecting the thatch. Another shortcoming is the need to replace the roof every two to three years because thatch deteriorates quickly. The second method of roofing involves the use of imported corrugated steel sheets. These last 10 years, do not involve a great deal of collection time, and are waterproof. They unfortunately cost more than one year's income; therefore, only a few people can afford them.

By identifying factors as illustrated in the last paragraph, the health care worker can catalogue building options and select the best material for the job. Alternative materials should also be explored. The use of metal roofs in rural Liberia is a recent practise, but is growing in popularity because of the material's durability.

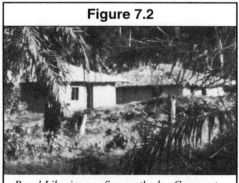

Figure 7.2

Rural Liberian roofing methods. Corrugated metal roof is used for the hut on the left while the right hut uses thatch.

Creativity also plays a role in applying available materials in a non-traditional fashion. The old saying, One person's junk is another person's treasure aptly describes the situation in developing countries. Since so few raw materials exist, every scrap of garbage is scavenged and used in some novel way. When an automobile can no longer be repaired, the car is stripped clean. Most of the sheet metal from the car will go into other metal projects such as a coal pot cook-stove. Even bald tires will be cut up and made into sandals. Metal cans are re-used for numerous projects. Nails are never discarded until they break into small pieces from repeated use. The watchful observer can note the ingenious ways community members find to recycle raw materials and adapt them to fit their own needs.

Transportation methods

It is often necessary to transport supplies or personnel from one location to another. Transportation options in LDCs are limited. Imagination must be used in identifying alternatives. Fossil-fuel-powered vehicles may be prohibitively expensive to maintain and operate. Animal- and human-powered vehicles may be the most appropriate alternative.

1. Cars and trucks
The method of transportation that is most obvious to a Westerner is by petrol-powered car or truck. This method requires no human labour, is fast, and can transport large amounts of materials and people. Unfortunately, it is unreliable (Figure 7.3). Poor road conditions and vehicle breakdowns are common. Secondly, it is expensive. Fuel and spare parts are costly. Identify locally available vehicles and question their owners about hiring options. If no vehicles exist in the project community then search surrounding towns for other options.

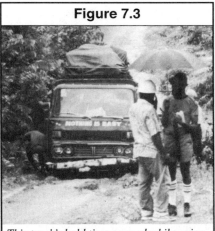

Figure 7.3

This truck's bald tires popped while going over a log bridge. There was no spare tire.

Given the poor roads, the lack of transportation methods and the paucity of health care facilities, many deaths occur because transportation is not available when illness strikes. Identify taxi drivers or other car operators who are willing to transport sick people on short notice to health care facilities for a set price. If this is not an option, then search for alternative methods of transportation as discussed below.

2. Human-powered transportation

Walking is as old as mankind and is still a viable transportation method. It is the most used mode of transportation in developing countries. When other methods fail, walking serves as a backup. Because walking is so slow and labour-intensive, other human-powered methods have evolved.

The bicycle greatly increases a person's range. It is cheaper than fuel based transportation options, and has fewer moving parts to break down. Although inexpensive, bicycles are too costly for most peasants. In addition, the amount that can be carried is limited. This has resulted in modifications to increase a bicycle's carrying capacity (Figure 7.4). Some bicycles become a cart with pedals while others have a carriage attached. This can allow the carrying of produce to market or the transportation of a sick person to a medical facility.

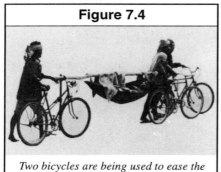

Figure 7.4

Two bicycles are being used to ease the burden of transporting a sick woman to a local clinic. Source: [6].

Human-powered carts are another transportation option that have been available for years. The rickshaw is one well-publicized example. Carts are also used for transporting food and other goods. They increase the carrying capacity, but still demand a large expenditure of human energy.

The main drawback to human-powered locomotion is the large input of manpower required. This caloric drain may have deleterious consequences on an already malnourished individual. It may still be the best option available, and may be most appropriate given limited resources. For people who always walk and carry supplies, a simple cart may actually decrease the workload and increase productivity.

3. Animal-powered transportation

An animal can generate more power, work for a longer time, and carry a larger load than a human. They cannot generate as much energy as a petrol-powered engine, but they are less likely to break down. They also are not dependent upon foreign fuels and parts. The health care worker should identify all animals in the community and assess their usefulness for transportation. Cultural factors will prevent the use of some animals as beasts of burden.

4. Water transportation

Rivers, lakes and oceans may provide an alternative transportation route to that of poorly maintained roads. For people who have lived around water all their lives, water transportation is probably already used. People who have recently moved near water may not appreciate its use as a transportation method. Nearby bodies of water and any local use of the water should be noted.

If people do not use water transport, then introduction of the concept may be helpful. For those who routinely travel on water, it may be possible to improve upon the current method. This often involves improved boat design, introduction of new methods to power the craft (e.g. sails, outboards) or opening up new waterways to extend the range of travel. As discussed previously, any change in the use of and exposure to water must occur only after careful consideration of the risk of water-borne diseases.

D. Alternative energy sources

People in developing countries expend a great deal of energy just staying alive. They rely on traditional labour-intensive methods to perform the required work. If alternative available energy sources can be identified and harnessed, the productivity and probably the health of the community will improve.

1. Humans and animals

These two groups supply the majority of energy for daily living in developing countries. Humans cannot produce large quantities of energy when compared to animals or engines. Man's advantage comes with the use of tools and machinery. Once labour-intensive tasks are identified, solutions that increase the efficiency of human work can be sought.

Women spend hours threshing and milling grain by hand for the evening meal. The introduction of appropriate technology can ease their burden by decreasing the work involved. A foot-operated thresher may be more efficient than beating the grain stalks with sticks (Figure 7.5). A hand mill may turn a two-hour task of pounding the grain with a mortar and pestle into a 15-minute job (Figure 7.6). The health care worker must identify where and how people expend their energy. This provides an estimate of the human power available, and can suggest ways to utilize that energy better.

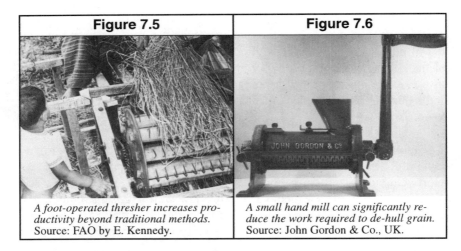

Figure 7.5: *A foot-operated thresher increases productivity beyond traditional methods.* Source: FAO by E. Kennedy.

Figure 7.6: *A small hand mill can significantly reduce the work required to de-hull grain.* Source: John Gordon & Co., UK.

Animals are the major energy producer in many rural communities. The numbers and types of animals in the community should be noted. The tasks they perform are also important and can suggest ways to improve their usefulness. Figure 7.7 illustrates the novel use of a horse or donkey to grind grain [1].

2. Electricity and fossil fuels

The availability of electricity and petrol should be ascertained. Since these energy types usually depend on imported equipment and supplies, an idea of their daily and year-round availability must be gained. It is not uncommon to have electricity and petrol available for only part of a day or for only certain times of the year. The cost of using electricity and petrol is important at the project level and at the community level. If a hospital is dependent upon a constant supply of electricity, but it does not generate enough income to pay for the electricity, the hospital will be without this energy source most of the time. This limits such essentials as vaccine refrigerators, centrifuges, X-rays, etc.

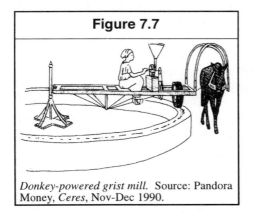

Figure 7.7: *Donkey-powered grist mill.* Source: Pandora Money, *Ceres*, Nov-Dec 1990.

3. Natural energy sources

Sunlight, water and wind are natural energy sources that have been harnessed for centuries and offer promise for future generations. They are non-polluting and relatively inexhaustible. With careful planning, they can supply some of the needed energy.

Solar power. Sunlight has many uses and many ways of being harvested. When abundant sunlight exists, as is often the case for many developing countries, it can be used to heat water, or to heat homes. Solar ovens can be constructed out of simple materials. They do function, but are slow. The Pax World Foundation [2] is developing a solar water purification device which harnesses the sun's energy to facilitate the purification process. The warmth of the sun can dry food for storage. Photovoltaic solar panels provide an opportunity for rural health posts to have uninterrupted electricity all year round. They have shown promise in powering high-efficiency vaccine refrigerators [3,4] (Figure 7.8).

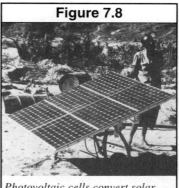

Figure 7.8

Photovoltaic cells convert solar energy to electricity. Source: FAO by J. von Dohnany.

From the most basic use of the sun to the high tech world of solar panels, the sun provides alternate energy options. The health care worker can measure the availability of sunlight from personal experience as well as from climactic charts. Based on this, one can apply known technologies to harness the sun's energy.

Water power. Rivers and streams represent another form of energy that can be harvested. Small waterfalls can turn waterwheels which then power machinery. Water-powered mills can ease a woman's workload by grinding grains into flour. Where appropriate, micro-hydroelectric plants can be installed to provide electricity for small cities or factories. Although the number of streams with enough vertical drop to run machinery may be small, their use should be explored.

Wind power. The use of wind may be more applicable than that of water. Many less developed countries are arid. Therefore, water is in short supply, while the barren environment provides ample wind to power machinery. Wind can provide power in a variety of ways and can perform many common tasks. A windmill can raise water from a well so that hand-pumping is not necessary. Windmills can power small mills for grinding grain. Windmills can also power turbines to generate electricity (Figure 7.9).

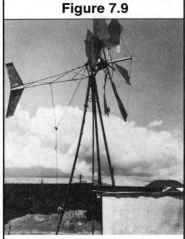

Figure 7.9

Windmills can pump water, run mills, or generate electricity. Source: FAO by E. Kennedy.

Harvesting natural energy sources requires a significant technological and monetary investment that is beyond the reach of most poor Third World communities. These high-cost projects may still have a role to play because of their renewable nature. If foreign agencies can provide the initial capital, the interventions may become self sustaining. Projects which have a lower initial cost but require moderate sums of money every month may cost more in the long run.

Powering vaccine refrigerators is one example where long-range planning may pay off. Vaccine refrigerators can be powered with mains electricity, fossil fuels like paraffin*, or by 12-volt DC current. The cost of a refrigerator does not vary much between models that are powered differently. When comparing the cost of equipping a rural clinic with a paraffin refrigerator or with a solar-powered refrigerator, the kerosene option will be cheaper initially since solar panels and batteries are quite expensive. Over time though, the paraffin refrigerator may be more expensive. A constant supply of paraffin must be available and must be purchased while the solar panel will provide electricity for at least 10 years. Given the cost of paraffin and the cost of spoiled vaccines due to periods of paraffin shortage, the solar-powered vaccine refrigerator will be less costly after 10 years of operation.

With judicious use, natural energy sources can meet some of the energy needs of developing countries. Traditional practises may rely on these natural energy sources. They should be identified and encouraged. Once an estimate of available natural energy is obtained, interventions can be structured to draw on these renewable energies.

Monetary and material resources

Interventions require money and materials. Ideally, these resources should come from the community the interventions are meant to help. Sustainable projects depend upon the constant input of resources. When com-

---

* i.e. kerosene.

munity resources fall short of those required to maintain a project, the project will fail [5]. The monetary and material worth of the average citizen must be assessed. Interventions should be based on these facts.

Published statistics exist for the average income of people living in selected less developed countries. Personal observation of people's livelihood can add to the information obtained from the literature. Observing what people buy and what they own can provide clues to personal economic freedom.

In many cases, morbidity and mortality are inversely related to family income. Therefore, assessing a family's financial means can provide an indirect estimate of their risk of ill health. For a family with limited financial reserves, one unfortunate event can ruin the family.

The death of a family's ox results in not only the loss of their one valuable possession, but also means there is no way to work the land. The family will be unable to make a living, or will go hopelessly into debt with the acquisition of a new animal. A major illness of a family member can result in large medical bills. This may necessitate the selling of the ox, or of incurring a huge debt. If the ill family member is the major income earner, the double effect of no income and increased expenditure may result in the disintegration of the family.

Estimating a family's monetary resources is important at both the individual and community level. A family with some reserves can tolerate minor health and financial setbacks. A community composed of families that possess some money, tools and materials will be likely to begin and sustain a community project. Quantifying these resources often requires the identification of indicator possessions.

In many cultures it is inappropriate to ask about family income. People may also fear that they will incur higher taxes if the family's actual income is known. This can lead to under-reporting of income and assets. The use of questions which indirectly ask about income may be more helpful in estimating a family's socioeconomic status. Questions like those listed in

Table 7.2
Indicator questions to estimate family wealth

Do your children attend school?
Do you have a radio or television?
Do you keep animals?
Do you have a refrigerator?

> **Community resources reduce project cost**
>
> In order to construct a health clinic, community members were required to make cement blocks by hand. One member supplied moulds for the blocks. Another member allowed the use of her shovel. A third member loaned some extra roofing material to shelter the workers and the bricks from the sun and the rain. Once the blocks were made, the tools and materials went back to their owners. Since these donated supplies did not have to be purchased, the monetary cost of the project was reduced.

Table 7.2 may produce a more accurate estimate of family income than asking a direct question about income. Families that own much are more likely to have a greater income than families that own nothing.

While observing what people own, one should catalogue spare building materials, equipment, machinery and tools. When the need arises, these materials or tools may be essential to completing a project. The owner of the resources should be asked to assist the project by supplying the needed materials (see box above).

By identifying resources that already exist in the community, interventions become more affordable and therefore possible.

Outside resources

When the money, resources and personnel are not available in the community, outside help must be sought. Perseverance and creativity are essential in locating outside help. The goods and services needed will dictate where to look for resources.

1. Money
Money is the most desired and scarce resource. Encouraging people or agencies to donate money requires much effort.

Many LDCs have foreign embassies in their capital city. These foreign governments may have self-help funds available. The funds are for community groups that are trying to improve their standard of living. Community members must make a written request to the foreign government in the form of a project proposal. Most self-help programmes require that the communities provide 25 percent of the total project cost. This 25 percent can be in the form of raw materials and labour. The maximum award amount varies with the embassy, but most self-help programmes rarely award more than £6,000 to one group.

Many foreign governments and consortia have development agencies whose purpose is to pursue large-scale interventions in developing countries. Examples are USAID and the EC. Both of these agencies are active in funding large projects. The United Nations has a number of branches which carry out similar development activities. These development agencies are geared more towards huge projects. Small communities are less likely to procure self-help funds. The community assessment site may fall within the boundaries of one of these large agencies' projects. Therefore, the community may be able to access some money or materials. The health care worker should check with the main office of these agencies.

Many church groups, private voluntary organizations and non-governmental organizations are active in Third World development projects. They sometimes provide money, personnel, expertise, medicines, equipment or materials to communities. It is best to approach groups that are already active in the host country.

Community groups may borrow money from local banks. This approach demands particular attention to the community's ability to pay back the loan, and is best used for projects that will generate income. For a community to borrow money, it must be well organized, and significant amounts of resources must already exist in the community. The proposed project must have a high probability of success and the community members must understand the consequences if the project fails.

2. Personnel
When skilled workers are needed but cannot be located in the target community, other regions must be searched. Skilled workers tend to congregate in cities. Craft guilds or worker's unions may exist that can direct the health worker to reputable craftspeople. Universities and schools are excellent places to locate people with special skills. Agricultural and rural development ministries may also provide information about people who can meet the project's needs.

Care must be exercised when using outside help, since their commitment to the community's well-being may be minimal. It is best to define clearly and in written form what is expected of the workers and how much they will be paid for their work. How to deal with workers will in part be controlled by cultural norms. In some societies it is best to pay the workers only after certain parts of the job have been completed. If the worker is paid the entire amount up front, the worker may never complete the task and disappear with the community's money. For example, if a mason has been hired to construct the walls of a building, the mason should be paid a small fee to get started. Once the foundation is completed, the mason will be paid for the work. When the walls are up, the mason will be paid for that work. When the job is complete, the final sum agreed upon will be given to the mason. This should be explicit in the contract. In this way, both parties get what they expect.

3. Books and educational materials

Health education is a major component of primary health care. The process of health education is enhanced when educational materials are present. Many of the agencies listed above in the money section have educational materials. Other groups such as TALC (Teaching Aids at Low Cost) and World Neighbors offer books, slides, filmstrips, etc. that were designed for people in developing communities. UNICEF and WHO have large selections of educational materials. These companies and organizations sell the materials at low cost.

Since people in different cultures learn in different ways, educational materials must be adapted to local needs. In one culture, the colour red may signify danger while in another culture the colour red may mean that all is well. If an educational poster that uses colours to convey a message is used in these two communities, the message conveyed will be quite different. When educational materials that were developed for other cultures are used, the materials must be altered to fit the new culture.

Summary. Identifying community resources is an essential part of community assessment. People are the most valuable resource a community has, but raw materials, power supplies and money are also necessary components. After targeting health problems, available resources can be used to combat the causes of ill health.

References

1. *Ceres* No. 126, Vol. 22, No. 2, Nov-Dec 1990:6.
2. The Pax World Foundation, 4400 East West Highway, Suite 130, Bethesda, MD 20814
3. Immunization. *Health Technology Directions*;9(2). Seattle: Program for Appropriate Technology in Health, 1989.
4. WHO, (1985). Expanded Programme on Immunization: Solar Powered Refrigerators for Vaccine Storage and Icepack Freezing: Status Summary June 1985. Geneva, WHO:28.
5. Bossert T. J., (1990). 'Can They Get Along Without Us? Sustainability of Donor-Supported Health Projects in Central America and Africa', *Soc. Sci. Med.*, 30(9):1015-1023.
6. Williams C. D., Baumslag N., Jelliffe D. B., (1985). '*Mother and Child Health: Delivering the Services*', Oxford University Press, Second Edition:23.

Chapter 8

Health, health care and endemic diseases

The goal of community assessment, as it relates to health, is to identify common illnesses, identify people at risk of ill health, and estimate access to health care. The health care worker must employ an eclectic approach to answer these questions. The purpose of obtaining this information is to focus interventions which aim to improve health.

Since a common theme for all developing countries is a lack of resources, it is necessary to target high-risk groups and identify the illnesses that afflict them. Limited resources can then be targeted at those people who most need them. This results in the greatest improvements in health while using the smallest amount of resources. Women and children represent the largest group at risk of serious illness. In addition, they have the poorest access to health care. Other at-risk groups exist because of certain endemic diseases or harmful lifestyles. Their access to health care may be blocked by many physical and cultural barriers. By identifying these at-risk groups, community assessment will realize its greatest impact.

Answers to the questions in Table 8.1 will guide the health care worker in assessing the health needs of the community. Both published literature and on-site evaluations should be used to answer these questions. The questions are the basis of descriptive epidemiology.

Table 8.1	
What health services exist?	What are the common illnesses, and are they treatable?
Who has access to these services?	
Where are the services located?	When does illness occur?
When are the services available?	Where does illness occur?
Why are services not available?	Why does illness occur?
Who needs these services?	

Health care availability

Locating available health care services may be easy. Determining the level of services offered and identifying those who have access to these services is more difficult. The published literature, ministries of health and district health managers can guide health care workers to recognized health care facilities. Determining accessibility and coverage requires knowledge of community demographics, economics and culture. In addition to Western medical services, an effort should be made to locate traditional healers and estimate their efficacy in meeting the health needs of the community.

Published literature is the first place to search for health care availability. Statistics taken from *The State of the World's Children 1990* regarding the Niger reveal that 41 percent of Niger's people have access to some form of health care. Ninety-nine percent of city dwellers have access while only 30 percent of rural dwellers have access. It is common for large segments of a developing country's population to lack access to Western health care. In addition, city dwellers have better access than rural dwellers. In fact, in some poor countries, a child living in a rural area only has a 10 percent chance of ever seeing a health care professional [1]. From this it can be seen that the current health care structure is not meeting the needs of the people (See box below).

Maldistribution of health care resources

The entire budget of low-income countries is very small in comparison to developed, industrialized nations. Third World governments often direct limited resources away from health and education toward military expenditures. Therefore, the health care budgets in these countries is understandably limited. Maldistribution of resources occurs even within the health care system. A large percentage of the health care budget is directed to serve urban-based politicians and urban elite. The result has been the construction of large curative-based city hospitals which serve these special interest groups, but neglect the much larger rural poor group. In Ghana, 85 percent of the health care budget is used by hospitals which treat 10 percent of the population. The remaining 15 percent of the money is directed to primary care which provides for 90 percent of the population [2].

Imbalance in present health care expenditure

Primary health care	Specialized health care
• Low cost	• Expensive
• Difficult to introduce	• Easy to introduce
• Great effect on common health problems	• Prestigious
	• Little effect on health problems

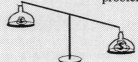

Source: Modified from D. Werner and M. Blake, *Helping Health Workers Learn*, Hesperian Foundation, PO Box 1692, Palo Alto, CA 94302, USA.

By locating national and regional statistics, the health care worker can gain an understanding of what facilities are available, where they are located and who has access to them. Direct observation and questioning at the community level will provide an estimate of the local availability of health care.

1. Barriers to health care

Many reasons exist for underutilization of health services. A patient's perceived need for medical care is considered the most important determinant of health care utilization. Factors like distance to the nearest clinic and family income also alter utilization patterns. Individual and family characteristics such as age, sex, family size, educational level and religious beliefs are other determinants of health facility use. The type of available health care and the perceived quality of health care contributes to utilization. All of these factors can be barriers to health care use. Since these barriers are interrelated in a complex fashion that researchers have yet to untangle, it may prove more effective for the health care worker to begin by estimating the percentage of the population that uses the available health care. If a cursory examination of utilization rates suggests that many people are not using the available health services, the health worker can then focus on the common barriers to health care.

The easiest way to estimate utilization rates is to rely on available data. If population size and clinic visit rates are available, an estimate for utilization rates may be gained. If one clinic serves a population of 10 000, but there are only 200 patient visits to the clinic per month, either the population is very healthy (unlikely), or people find health care barriers insurmountable.

Since such an extreme case as illustrated above is unlikely, other methods of estimating health care utilization are necessary. It may be helpful to follow health care utilization for only one disease. Although health care utilization is partially dependent on the type of illness a person has, when survey capabilities are limited, this indicator disease may be the most appropriate method of estimating health care use.

In areas where an estimate of the prevalence of an endemic disease is available, this endemic disease may be useful as an indicator illness. For example, if the monthly incidence of malaria in a community of 10 000 inhabitants is estimated at five percent, the average number of new cases local clinics treat should be about 500. If the number of people treated for malaria each month by the clinics is significantly less than 500, utilization, or coverage, is said to be poor. If several endemic diseases can be used as indicator diseases, then the estimate of utilization is more likely to be accurate. Because utilization varies with the type of illness, following more than one illness will reduce the risk of skewed results due to a poor selection of indicator disease.

When demographic and clinic records are not available, and the resources for a survey are inadequate, the health care worker will have to rely on observation and casual questioning of local inhabitants. This method is time-consuming and the potential for error is significant, but with care, useful and accurate information can be obtained.

Medical anthropologists use observation and questioning effectively to collect information about communities. One simple anthropological method involves the questioning of key informants. A few community members are selected who are then questioned at length. Their answers can give a general idea of prevalent beliefs. For example, information can be gathered regarding which illnesses are perceived as being better treated by traditional or Western methods. The key informant method is liable to biased views of a community, but it may also uncover information that a more traditional epidemiological survey would miss.

Once utilization is found to be less than expected, through observation and questioning or scrutiny of available data, the health care worker should then focus on potential barriers. Once barriers are identified, the hope is that the health care worker will remove the significant ones.

Perceived need. A patient's perceived need of health care services is the most important determinant of utilization [3-5]. In a study by Fosu (1989), perceived need at the household level was found to account for 69 percent of clinic use [6]. This effect of perceived need on health care utilization is intuitive. If a person does not perceive they are sick, then of course there would be no need to seek health care. The perception of being sick depends on many factors. Fosu found that as the number of medical conditions a person suffered increased and as the time ill increased, the community member was more likely to use available health care. O. S. Habib and J. P. Vaughan (1986) found that utilization, or perceived need, also depended on the type of illness [7]. Although respiratory diseases accounted for 21.6 percent of reported illness, and infectious or parasitic diseases accounted for only seven percent of illness, health care use was much greater for people with parasitic or infectious diseases (111.0 versus 79.3 consultations per 100 episodes). Care must be taken with these findings since perceived need is influenced by many other factors including cultural and religious beliefs.

Distance. Many studies have demonstrated that as distance to a health clinic increases, utilization of health services decreases (Figure 8.1) [7-10]. An understanding of the population size and density is necessary to estimate accessibility. In general, a health facility is accessible if a person can get there in approximately two hours of travel. This is a six-mile walk for the average person and a variable distance for someone travelling by other means. Travel times in excess of two hours will reduce the chance of people presenting for routine health care. Many people will only make the journey when they are seriously ill.

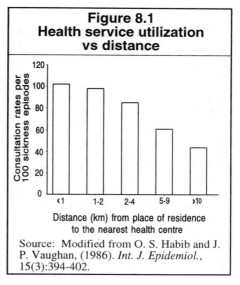

**Figure 8.1
Health service utilization vs distance**

Source: Modified from O. S. Habib and J. P. Vaughan, (1986). *Int. J. Epidemiol.*, 15(3):394-402.

Perceived quality of health care. Even when a health centre is only a short distance away, barriers may exist which limit access. If the clinic is short staffed and busy, the average wait to be seen may be too long. A long wait has been shown to decrease immunization coverage [11,12]. The health care that is provided may be seen as unacceptably poor [13]. Patients may be treated with disrespect by the health facility staff, or patients may be threatened by the sterile Western medical environment. Pharmaceuticals may be unavailable most of the time. Community members may prefer to use traditional healers. In some situations this may be appropriate. All of these factors can decrease the percentage of people who use an available health care facility.

Cost. Cost is a major obstacle to accessing health care. Because resources are so limited, many health care facilities require payment in full before treatment begins. If the person cannot pay, then treatment is not given. The very poor may find even subsidized clinic costs exorbitant and seek health care from traditional healers or drug stores. Utilization of health services generally increases with increasing family income (Figure 8.2). In communities where multiple health facilities exist, wealthier families

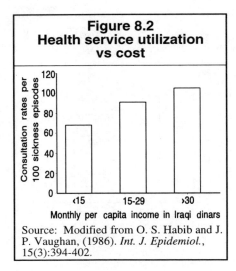

Figure 8.2
Health service utilization vs cost

Source: Modified from O. S. Habib and J. P. Vaughan, (1986). *Int. J. Epidemiol.*, 15(3):394-402.

may choose to use private practitioners and avoid cheaper public clinics. This factor could decrease the perceived utilization of health services.

Inquiries should be made regarding the fee schedule for the primary health care facility and the referral health care facility. From this, the affordability in the eyes of the community members can be estimated. If people cannot afford the prices, then utilization will be less.

Social factors. Many social factors will affect health care utilization. For sensitive topics like birth control and family planning, religious beliefs may dictate whether a person can visit a health facility. The parents of an unwed pregnant teenager from a devout Muslim or Christian family might deny their daughter access to a clinic for fear of shaming the family. Muslim women will often not attend a clinic that has only male providers. An Animist may feel a traditional healer is better able to cure their illness than would a Western-trained health care professional.

Educational level is another potential barrier to health care access. The lower the educational level of the head of the household, the lower the access rate of the family to available health care. This observation may be obscured as community members patronize traditional healers, drug stores, public or private clinics.

2. Health facility services

Once the health care facility is identified, the health worker should evaluate the breadth of services offered. Is the health facility a community health worker's post that has limited availability of medicines and no invasive procedure capabilities; or is the health facility a missionary hospital with extensive operative and diagnostic facilities? If the health facility is unable to treat common life-threatening illnesses, questions should be asked regarding referral facilities. Especially for obstetric complications, there is a need for rapid and reliable transportation to a referral facility that has operative capabilities [14,15]. Gaining an understanding of available referral facilities and transportation methods is important in understanding the level of available health care.

The physical existence of a health facility does not guarantee health care. Some facilities operate only intermittently or routinely run out of essential supplies including medications. If a health centre has only a limited number of providers, illness or absence of a health worker may result in the temporary closure of the facility. Many clinics in developing countries, even in major cities, lack electrical power and running water. Even when these services are available, they may be intermittent at best. If this is the case, long periods may occur where diagnostic and surgical capabilities are not available.

Many health care workers in developing countries have learned that without supplies and medicines, very few curative services can be offered. A community health worker may be able to diagnose pneumonia, but if the antibiotics necessary to treat the child are unavailable or are not affordable, the child may die of the infection. The visiting health care worker needs to identify locally available medicines and gain an appreciation for their cost in relation to the income of the average local inhabitant. Questions should be asked regarding year-round availability of medicines [16].

3. Essential medicines

WHO has proposed the use of an essential drug list by less developed countries as a way of combating the persistent problem of drug shortages (Table 8.2) [17,18]. This plan is based on the fact that a majority of people get sick with a limited number of common diseases. For a common infection like pneumonia, 20 different types of antibiotics are not needed. It is more cost-effective to have only one or two different antibiotics available for all health care workers to treat this common infection. In this way exotic (i.e. expensive) medicines are not purchased, and only one brand name of each medicine is procured.

An essential medications list may be composed of only 100 to 150 drugs. For each class of drug (e.g. penicillin) only one brand is purchased. In this way, a country can buy medicines in bulk from one manufacturer at a discounted rate for use in the entire country. Countries often accept bids from reputable pharmaceutical companies and then select the lowest offer. This not only saves money by buying in bulk, but also decreases the cost of importation. An essential medicines programme allows the majority of people in a community to have medicines always available to treat their

Table 8.2
Example of an essential antibiotics list

Medicine	Unit	Cost(U.S. $)	Cost/Dose
Ampicillin caps 250mg	1000	$24.00	$0.03
Amp powder 125mg/ml	60 ml	$0.35	$0.01
Amp inj. 500mg/ amp	100 amps	$12.31	$0.13
Chloramphenicol caps 250mg	1000	$18.21	$0.02
Chloramphenicol inj, vial	25	$7.50	$0.03
Co-trimoxazole tabs 400/80	1000	$31.27	$0.03
Co-trimoxazole syrup 200/40/5cc	1	$1.29	$1.29
Erythromycin tabs 250mg	1000	$28.62	$0.03
Gentamicin inj 80mg/ml	25	$4.29	$0.17
PenVK tabs 250mg	1000	$12.79	$0.02
Procaine PCN 10cc	100	$21.54	$0.22
Tetracycline caps 250mg	1000	$9.13	$0.01

Source: Taken from the essential medicines list for Sinoe County, Liberia

most common ailments. When specialty medicines are needed, the patient may turn to private pharmacies or be referred to major urban hospitals.

Revolving drug fund. Closely related to an essential medicines programme is the concept of a revolving drug fund [19]. Either a community, agency or government purchases a large quantity of essential medicines. After the initial purchase, no outside agency or group need place more money into purchasing medicines. When individuals purchase revolving fund medications, the money from the sale is then used to purchase replacement drugs. This describes the revolving nature of the resources from cash to drugs then back to cash so that the cycle can continue with another purchase of drugs.

The price of medicines for individual use is dependent upon the price paid for the entire essential medicines purchase. The price charged to the individual for a five day course of treatment will just pay for the cost of the medicine, plus a small overhead fee, but no additional profit will be made. In this way, the cost is reduced to the end user. A well-managed revolving drug fund can effectively provide essential medicines at an affordable cost. In effect, the middle business person is removed from the loop, thereby passing on significant savings to the ill patient.

A number of trouble spots exist in creating and maintaining a revolving drug fund. If local pharmacy owners have clout in the community, they may block the introduction of the revolving drug fund because it will decrease their sales. If unscrupulous health care workers or government officials skim money from the fund, the fund is sure to fail. Less capital will be available to purchase the next shipment of medicines. This results in increased cost to the patient or a decrease in the selection of available drugs. Some health care workers charge their own price for the revolving drugs in order to make extra income. This makes the medicines less affordable for the average user. Pilfering or loss of a shipment of essential medicines means the resources to maintain the drug fund are gone. New resources must be added to the fund, or the fund will cease. If the price of medicines on the world market increases, the cost to the user may rise above their ability to pay. Finally, if patients are given medicines on credit, it is difficult to collect these debts at a later date.

Even with the many potential pitfalls, a revolving drug fund is a viable solution to the problems of chronic shortages and high costs of medicines. Assessment of drug availability is a necessary part of defining the accessibility of health care services. If medicines are in short supply, an essential medicines list and a revolving drug fund may represent a possible solution.

4. Vertical programmes
In addition to ongoing curative services, many vertical programmes fill certain needs. Because of their intermittent nature, these programmes can be difficult to document during short-term assessment projects. Examples of these programmes include vaccination campaigns and health education teams. Ministry of health employees and health personnel in the project area may provide clues to intermittent services. Published literature can also help. In a country such as Niger where the population's access to health care is 40 percent, but 70 percent of children have received their basic immunizations, children must have been reached by some other mechanism. Further investigative work is then needed to identify possible intermittent vertical programmes.

Summary. By combining information from published literature and firsthand observation, the question of health care availability can be answered. Quantifying population size and number of health care facilities determines accessibility. Identifying factors that limit health care delivery provides an estimate of coverage. Knowledge about accessibility and coverage answer questions regarding the who, what, when, where and why of health care availability. With this information, effective interventions can be implemented.

At-risk groups

Within every community there are groups at greater risk of illness. These at-risk groups are also less likely to receive care for their illness. The health care worker needs to identify these high-risk groups and assess the opportunities they have for treatment. Predisposing factors for illness must also be recognized if any hope for change is to be realized. Once these at-risk groups are identified, limited resources can be directed to meet their health needs.

WHO has identified a major at-risk group by declaring maternal child health (MCH) a priority problem. Women and children are the largest oppressed group in the world. By observing a culture's prevalent attitude toward women, one can gain an appreciation for the potential health risks. If a woman is prized for her childbearing and work potential, it is generally true that she will be oppressed and neglected. If she is not allowed to vote or to own land, she is likely to be treated as a second class citizen in other areas of life.

1. Women

A number of indicators can be gleaned from the literature that direct a health care worker to the problems a woman faces in her culture. Table 8.3 presents common statistics which highlight certain risks for both women and children.

Bearing children. Women face the greatest risk to their health from childbearing. As can be seen from the maternal mortality ratio (MMR) for Rwanda, 210 women die for every 100 000 live births. Up to 15 times this number suffer significant morbidity [20]. Comparing the MMR statistic

Table 8.3
Indicators of women's health - Rwanda

Total fertility rate (TFR)	8.3
Female/male literacy rate	54%
Female/male secondary school enrollment	71%
Contraceptive prevalence	10%
Percent of pregnant women immunized against tetanus	43%
Percent of births attended by trained attendant	22%
Maternal mortality ratio(MMR)	210*

Source: UNICEF, (1990). *The State of the World's Children 1990.*
* 210 deaths per 100 000 live births.

with that of developed countries where the MMR is in the 5-15 range, one can see the great risk women face in bearing children (Figure 8.3). One study from The Gambia revealed that women in the study population had a MMR of over 1 000 [21].

Many reasons exist for this high MMR. One factor is the total number of children a woman has during her reproductive life. In Rwanda, where an average woman bears eight children (TFR = 8.3), her risk will be great. A high total fertility rate corresponds with a culturally approved view of women as baby factories. A woman's main worth is measured by the total number of children she can bear. Not only does a woman have too many children, but she also begins childbearing when she herself is still a child. In addition, she has children spaced too closely together, and has children for too long. These factors work synergistically to create the high maternal mortality ratio.

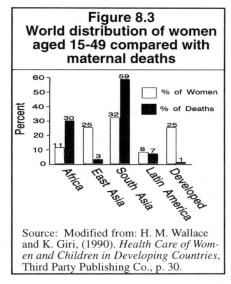

Figure 8.3
World distribution of women aged 15-49 compared with maternal deaths

Source: Modified from: H. M. Wallace and K. Giri, (1990). *Health Care of Women and Children in Developing Countries*, Third Party Publishing Co., p. 30.

Considering this high fertility rate along with the low percentage of women who deliver with the aid of a trained birth attendant (Figure 8.4), one gains an appreciation for why the MMR may be so high. Women are generally less mobile, have fewer resources, and are often dependent upon men for access to health care. The low prevalence of contraceptive usage supports this view. Inadequate access to health care professionals and contraceptive supplies limits access to birth control options. At least for countries in Sub-Saharan Africa, cultural practises also impinge upon contraceptive use. Large families are

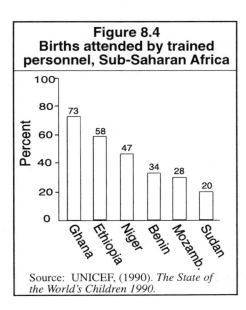

Figure 8.4
Births attended by trained personnel, Sub-Saharan Africa

Source: UNICEF, (1990). *The State of the World's Children 1990.*

still desired in Africa. A woman's worth is measured by her ability to bear children. Subsequently, the demand for contraception is low. The percent reduction in family size if a woman could stop having children when she wanted was estimated by one study to be 17 percent in Africa, 33 percent in Asia and 35 percent in Latin America [22]. Although the percentage is low in Africa, it still reveals that women do not have access to contraceptive methods that they desire.

Breast-feeding is the most natural form of child spacing and has a significant impact on family size. Unfortunately, breast-feeding is decreasing both in prevalence and duration [23-25]. This decrease is attributed to the introduction of Western ideas, urbanization, an increase in women entering the workforce and the marketing pressure applied by formula manufacturers [26]. In traditional societies, women normally breast-feed their babies for two to three years. As can be seen from Figure 8.5, this is no longer true. Only in 3.6 percent of countries studied did women breast-feed their children for more than two years. The result has been an increase in the fertility rate.

Immunization. The low percentage of women immunized against tetanus (Table 8.3) is another indicator that women have poor access to health care. Less than 50 percent of women have received adequate immunization. This means that women are either not being seen by the health care system or vaccination opportunities are missed. Tetanus immunization of women will actually have its greatest effect on children, since neonatal tetanus only occurs in newborns whose mothers have not been vaccinated.

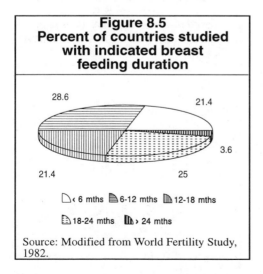

**Figure 8.5
Percent of countries studied with indicated breast feeding duration**

Source: Modified from World Fertility Study, 1982.

Education. Education of women is one of the few factors that has been linked to a significant improvement in the health of the family. As a woman's educational level improves, the health of her family improves. This has been found to be more important than even the level of household income [27]. Improving the level of education of men does not result in the same improvements in family health as does educating women. In Rwanda, male children receive more education than female children, and almost twice as many male children read as do female children (Table 8.3). In general, women are viewed as having less need for education because their main role in society is to stay in the home and care for children.

The health care worker does not have to perform a rigorous study to see if these statistics accurately represent the study population. Women can be asked about the number of children they have born, the approximate age when childbearing began, and the spacing between children. Sometimes this can simply be observed. The health care worker should also observe the role of women in society. When meeting with community leaders, if there are no women involved in the process, it suggests that women play a subservient role in that society. If women are seen mainly in the kitchen, noted to work hard all day, and are surrounded by many children, their worth is probably less than that of a man's. Asking questions about schooling and reading can provide clues as to the average educational level of women.

Observation of health care facilities and questioning health care workers will provide answers to health care availability for women. Are trained traditional birth attendants (TBAs) used? Where is the nearest health centre that has operative capabilities? Are contraceptives available locally, and are women trained in their use? Who decides when a woman can access health care? Answers to these questions provide insight into the problems women face.

2. Children
Children, like women, are vulnerable. Fortunately, they have received more attention than women. There remains much room for improvement. As previously stated, poor health and inadequate access to care for women translates into increased risk for children. As a woman's health deteriorates, she is less able to care for her children. The more work the mother must perform, the less time she will have available to care for her children. The less educated a woman, the less likely she is to try new ideas and to use available health care. Finally, she may have a more fatalistic view of life.

A number of statistical indicators exist in the literature that can direct the health care worker to problems which adversely affect children. Table 8.4 lists some important child health indicators.

Table 8.4
Indicators of children's health, Niger 1990

Under-five mortality rate (per 1000)	228
Infant mortality rate (per 1000)	134
Percent of age group in school	29%
Percent of infants with low birth weight	15%
Percent of mothers breast-feeding six-month-old children	30%
Percent of children moderately-severely underweight (up to four years)	49%
Calorie supply as percent of requirement	100%
Percent of population with access to safe water	47%
Percent of population with access to health care	41%
Oral rehydration soultion use rate	0.6%
Percent of immunized children	
TB	39%
DPT	16%
Polio	16%
Measles	24%
Maternal tetanus	8%

Source: UNICEF, (1990). *The State of the World's Children 1990.*

Children in low income countries are at high risk of dying prematurely. In Niger, nearly 25 percent of children born will never reach their fifth birthday. The average Niger woman will see two of the eight children she bore die before they reach their fifth birthday. From the Table it can be seen that over half of the 228 deaths occur in the first year of life because of an infant mortality rate of 134 per 1000 live births. In general, the younger the child the greater the risk of morbidity and early death [28]. If a child is fortunate enough to survive to school age, the risk of dying decreases significantly [29,30].

Figure 8.6 illustrates how precarious life is for the young in developing countries. Comparing the age at which death occurs for people in developed and developing countries, one can appreciate that death in developing countries occurs most often at younger ages. This fact suggests not only the time of life at which illness is most likely to occur, but also those who require the services.

The causes of the high under-five mortality rate are multifactorial. Birth-related events and infectious/parasitic diseases are the leading causes of death for children in developing countries. It is estimated that 3.2 million deaths, or 22 percent of all under-five deaths are due to perinatal causes. Infectious/parasitic maladies account for 10.5 million deaths, or 72 percent

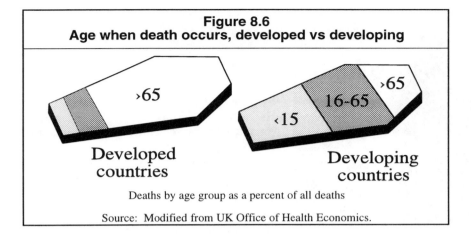

**Figure 8.6
Age when death occurs, developed vs developing**

Deaths by age group as a percent of all deaths

Source: Modified from UK Office of Health Economics.

of all under-five deaths. The only other significant cause of death in this age group is accidents or violence which contribute 6 percent, or 900 000 deaths per year [31].

Undernutrition and infection. The incidence of undernutrition remains unacceptably high (Table 8.5). Although not generally listed as a major cause of death, undernutrition works in concert with other illnesses to increase morbidity and mortality. Therefore, an infectious illness is more likely to be fatal for a malnourished child than for a well-fed child [32-35]. Not only does malnutrition increase the risk of death from infection, but infection can decrease food intake [36,37]. This interaction may result in a vicious cycle whereby infection predisposes a child to undernutrition and undernutrition increases the severity and complications of infection [38].

**Table 8.5
Estimates of annual cases of malnutrition in
children aged 0-4 years, by region 1973-1983**

Region	Millions	Percent
Africa	21.9	25.6
Asia	114.6	54.0
Latin America	8.6	17.1
Total	145.1	26.0

Source: Modified from 'Global Trends in Protein-Energy Malnutrition', *Bull. Pan. Amer. Hlth. Org.*, 18(4), 1984.

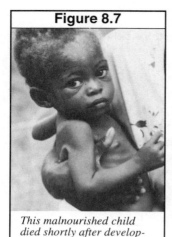

Figure 8.7

This malnourished child died shortly after developing diarrhoea.

Low birthweight greatly increases the chance of an early death (Figure 5.3). As stated previously, low birthweight in Third World children is generally a result of undernutrition in the mother and not to prematurity as is common in developed countries.

Malnutrition has deleterious effects on the immune system [39,40]. This results in a decreased ability to eradicate infections [41-44]. It has been shown that underweight children are more likely to have prolonged diarrhoea with a higher risk of complications than well-nourished children (Figure 8.7) [45-49]. Also, some studies suggest that diarrhoea has an adverse effect on growth [50-53]. Malnourished children who develop acute respiratory infections stay sick longer, experience greater severity of disease, and have a higher mortality than do well-nourished children [54,55]. Vitamin A deficiency has been linked to an increased mortality rate in children [56,57], especially in children with measles. Vitamin A deficiency is also associated with an increased risk of developing respiratory infections and diarrhoea [58].

Close to half of all children in Niger exhibit signs of moderate to severe undernutrition (Table 8.4). Maldistribution of food appears to be a significant cause since theoretically, Niger citizens are supplied with 100 percent of their caloric needs. This maldistribution of food may occur at all levels, from national to household. Indicators to assist the health care worker in identifying distribution problems were discussed in a previous section.

The health care worker can estimate the prevalence of under-five malnutrition in the community by measuring the mid upper arm circumference of children between the ages of 12-59 months. During this age range, the arm circumference is constant at about 16cm. A measurement below 12.5cm is a strong indicator of undernutrition. Although not as accurate as weight for age, arm circumference measurements require minimal equipment, can be performed by illiterate health care workers, and provide useful information about the general nutritional status of 12-59-month-old children in the community [59].

For brief visits to isolated areas, the health care worker can gain an appreciation of the prevalence of malnutrition in children by just feeling the size

Table 8.6
Estimates of major causes of death in children under 5

Cause	Estimated annual deaths
Dehydration due to diarrhoea	5 million
Pneumonia	3 million
Measles	2 million
Whooping cough	1.6 million
Neonatal tetanus	1 million
Malaria	750000
Poliomyelitis	50000
Diphtheria	5000

Source: WHO, 1985.

of children's arms. If the health care worker practises identifying the feel of a 12.5cm circumference arm, the worker can assess a child by just holding the child's mid upper arm. TALC sells model plastic arms of various circumferences so the health care worker can practise this simple measurement technique. If it is felt that malnutrition may be present in the community, a more exacting study can be carried out using measured arm circumference or weight-for-age measurements.

Among the diseases that adversely affect children diarrhoea, acute respiratory infections, vaccine-preventable illnesses and malaria (often ignored as a leading cause of death) are major contributors to premature death. Table 8.6 lists gross estimates of the number of deaths attributable to each malady. Unfortunately, an accurate assessment of these illnesses is often difficult. Hospital-based studies are not representative of the community. Community-based studies are expensive and often suffer from methodological flaws. This contributes to inaccuracy and limits comparability between studies [60].

Diarrhoea, dehydration and oral rehydration therapy (ORT). Inadequate sanitation, poor personal hygiene and a shortage of potable water are associated with an increased incidence of diarrhoea. The Niger data reveals that less than one half of the population has a safe water supply. In rural areas, the problem is greater. To date, interventions to prevent diarrhoea have been limited. Fortunately, ORT is an effective treatment for dehydration caused by diarrhoea.

Dehydration is the final common pathway for deaths due to diarrhoea. Therefore, ORT use is correlated with a decrease in deaths due to diar-

**Table 8.7
Percentage of health care professionals who are trained in ORS use.**

Physicians	14%
Nurses	4%
Paramedics	8%
Community health workers	9%

Source: WHO, 1988.

rhoea [61]. For the 60 countries with the highest under-five mortality rate, oral rehydration solution (ORS) use is under 12 percent [62]. Health care workers are partly to blame since many of them do not encourage the use of ORT (Table 8.7).

Because health care workers play an important role in teaching community members about ORT, an estimate of its use can be ascertained by questioning health care workers. If health professionals are unaware of the benefits of ORT and prefer to prescribe anti-diarrhoeal medicines and antibiotics, the chance of community members using ORT is small. However, in communities where vertical ORT educational programmes are carried out, there may be a poor correlation between health care worker's acceptance and ORT use rates.

The converse of the previous assumption is not necessarily true. In communities where ORT use is encouraged by health workers or vertical programmes, it cannot be assumed that ORT use is high. J. D. and D. S. Mull (1988) [63] found that in rural Pakistan, where a massive ORT education campaign took place over three years, 28 percent of respondents had never heard of ORT. Only 56 percent of the population studied ever used ORS. Of the 56 percent who used ORS, only 38 percent had any idea of how to prepare and administer the solution.

Besides decreasing mortality from dehydration, ORT decreases the cost of treating diarrhoea. Oral rehydration solution is less expensive than both IV hydration and ineffective medicines which are frequently used. As ORS use rate increases, expenditure on non-rehydration medicines decreases [64]. Given the limited per capita health care budget, an increase in ORT can increase the capital available for other health interventions.

Acute Respiratory Infections (ARI). Acute respiratory infections are a leading cause of death in children under-five. The average child in less developed countries experiences between three and six respiratory infections per year [65]. Up to four million children a year die from respiratory infections. Infants of up to six months are at the greatest risk of dying from ARIs. Bacterial pneumonia due to *H. influenza* and *S. pneumonia* are the major killers. Malnourished children and children with measles are at an increased risk of death due to ARIs [66].

Significant risk factors for developing acute respiratory infections include age less than six months, poor nutrition (both Protein Energy Malnutrition (PEM) and Vitamin A), bottle-feeding, overcrowding, poor housing, low birthweight (<2500gms), poor personal hygiene, tobacco abuse (including passive smoking) and indoor air pollution (often cooking fires) [67]. Lack of appropriate immunizations against measles, *B. pertussis*, TB and *H. influenza*, also increase the risk of ARI and morbidity [68].

Unlike ORS for the treatment of dehydration due to diarrhoea, there is no obvious quick fix remedy to decrease the mortality rate attributable to respiratory infections. The WHO has outlined a case-management scheme for the diagnosis and treatment of ARIs that is useful for health care workers to reduce the mortality associated with ARI effectively [69,70]. Ensuring appropriate and timely immunizations, encouraging breast-feeding and limiting exposure to air pollution may also decrease ARI-associated mortality by decreasing its incidence. For these interventions to work, area health care professionals must be well trained, have the proper equipment (e.g. cold chain), and have a constant supply of medications (antibiotics and vaccines).

Vaccination. It is difficult to assess both the immunization coverage rate and the prevalence of immunization-preventable diseases while carrying out a qualitative community survey. Published literature about vaccination coverage for a country is not applicable to specific communities in that country. National survey data may be inaccurate if actual sero-positive immunity was not measured. A child who is recorded as being immunized may have received a vaccine that was rendered inactive by prolonged exposure to heat. A number of follow-up studies have demonstrated that failures in the cold chain result in heat-inactivated vaccines being used at peripheral health posts [71,72]. Without the ability to check titres, the health care worker must rely on reports of vaccination activities in the community from project site members and local health workers.

Checking with a country's ministry of health or the staff of the district hospital may provide a starting point for estimating the coverage rate for immunizations. Questions posed should include: estimates of vaccination coverage rates by region/population, the availability and reliability of cold chain equipment, the prevalence of diseases preventable by immunizations, current methods for immunizing children and the occurrence of special vertical immunization campaigns.

If the prevalence rates for diseases preventable by immunization are high, coverage of the population in question must be low. This may result from a combination of factors. When only a low percentage of the population is adequately immunized, the protective effect of herd immunity* is absent. The use of vaccines that have been rendered ineffective by faulty cold chain techniques not only inadequately protects children, but also provides a false sense of security. Particularly virulent strains of the infectious agent can overcome the mildly protective effect of partial immunity.

If vaccination coverage rates (actual immunity) are low, further questioning is needed to uncover the causes. Cold chain problems often contribute to a low coverage rate [73]. Lack of vaccines may be another reason. More disconcerting is that 69 percent of children brought to health care clinics for non-immunization reasons, but who were in need of immunizations, did not receive any vaccines during the visit [74]. This missed opportunity by health care workers is a major contributor to low immunization rates. This is one area in which intervention requires simple education of health care workers and is not dependent upon expensive imported supplies.

The study population should be questioned about immunizations. It should be a common practise when immunizing children to give the mothers some record of the immunizations. If mothers have such records, coverage can be monitored and assessed. All children in each household must be identified and their immunization status questioned. It is not uncommon for male children to be presented for immunizations and female children to be excluded [75,76], although this varies between cultures [77]. This is particularly true when a fee is charged for vaccination. In other cases, a child may not be taken for immunization because of sickness, or a health care worker may inappropriately exclude a sick child from receiving immunizations. By asking questions at the household level, the health worker can estimate the accuracy of district vaccination reports, and possibly identify groups that are missed by current immunization efforts.

Malaria. With an estimated 2.6 billion people at risk of malaria infection worldwide, and at least one million deaths annually, malaria remains a major killer. Children under five account for 75 percent of the one million malaria-related deaths. Malaria infections adversely affect children even before birth. Pregnant women infected with the malaria parasite are more likely to give birth to low birthweight newborns. Consequently, this indi-

---

* Herd immunity occurs when a large percentage of the population is immune to a specific illness. This high level of immunity greatly decreases the risk of illness. In addition, if one person becomes infected, the risk of that person contacting a susceptible individual is small.

rectly increases the neonate's morbidity and mortality. The health risks to children cannot be fully surmised without examining the role malaria plays in the community.

The first step in estimating the impact malaria has on children in the target community is to identify if malaria infections are endemic. Many basic medical texts contain information identifying malaria endemic countries (Figure 8.8). A number of epidemiological studies exist in the literature that actually estimate the prevalence of malaria in particular communities. It is common for malaria prevalence to be 50 percent or higher [78,79].

Once in the community, questioning people generally confirms the existence of malaria. If literature on its prevalence does not exist for the target community, estimating spleen rates in children can provide useful information (See page 111). Local health care workers may also provide useful information. Observing a number of factors will allow the health care worker to gauge the risk of malaria-related morbidity and mortality.

Living near large bodies of standing water such as swamps and rice paddies that support *Anopheles* mosquito development will increase the likelihood of disease transmission. Given the mosquito's propensity to be active from dusk to dawn (nighttime), people who are active outside during this time are more likely to be infected. In many areas, malaria transmission is increased during the rainy season. People who sleep in unscreened areas or without bednets risk infection [79]. Pregnant women, especially primiparous women, who do not receive chloroquine prophylaxis have an increased risk of ill health for themselves and their foetus. The existence

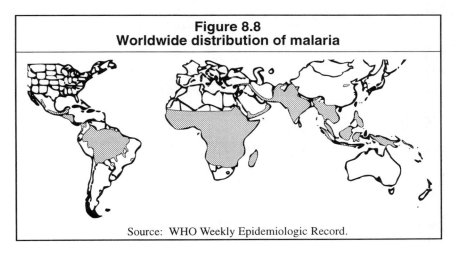

**Figure 8.8
Worldwide distribution of malaria**

Source: WHO Weekly Epidemiologic Record.

of chloroquine-resistant *falciparum* malaria greatly increases the risk of premature death in children. Lastly, the younger the child, the greater the risk of morbidity and mortality.

3. The elderly

An at-risk group that has recently gained more attention in the world is the geriatric sector. In comparison with developed countries, the elderly in LDCs make up a small proportion of the total population. They have thus far been neglected. This is unfortunate since their health care needs are great and their resources are limited. The plight of the elderly will worsen as the extended family structure continues to disintegrate.

The elderly are at significant risk of ill health. In a study from Kenya [80] it was found that 30 percent of elderly people lived alone, and a significant proportion (23 percent) did not own land. This suggests that the elderly are at risk of being isolated, and their income may be quite low (Figure 8.9). Their access to health care may be limited due to their low income, rural distribution, decreased mobility, traditional beliefs and cultural barriers.

The elderly living in rural areas experience a steady decline in height and weight (Figure 8.10). Malnutrition contributes to this. One potential indicator of undernutrition is the low haemoglobin levels seen in the elderly [81]. Waswa and others demonstrated that 21 percent of the individuals in their study were anaemic [80]. Most of those with low haemoglobin levels weighed less than 80 percent of the weight to be expected for their height. The elderly also experience an increase in the incidence of disease with advancing age. Oral disease and ocular problems appear to be significant maladies. With failing health, malnutrition, poor eyesight and limited resources, the elderly may be unable to care for themselves and may face a life of deprivation that ends prematurely.

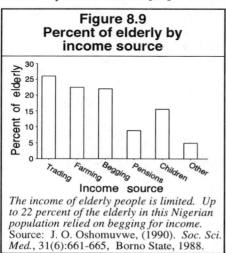

**Figure 8.9
Percent of elderly by income source**

The income of elderly people is limited. Up to 22 percent of the elderly in this Nigerian population relied on begging for income.
Source: J. O. Oshomuvwe, (1990). *Soc. Sci. Med.*, 31(6):661-665, Borno State, 1988.

4. Other at-risk groups
In addition to the high-risk groups mentioned above, each community will have other at-risk segments. Risk will depend upon such factors as residence, livelihood and lifestyle. Through simple observation, the health care worker can identify many of these groups.

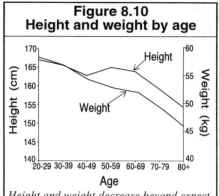

Figure 8.10
Height and weight by age

Height and weight decrease beyond expected values for age in the Kenyan male population studied. Source: J. K. Waswa, et al, (1988). *E. Afr. Med. J.*, 578-587, Sep.

Location. Where people live will in part dictate the types of illnesses they experience. For those communities located by fast-flowing streams, onchocerciasis (river blindness) may be a significant health problem. Those living by a swamp may find malaria and bilharziasis major causes of ill health. People who live in a major city may experience respiratory ailments due to air pollution. Location alone may suggest at-risk groups.

Occupational risks - trauma. A study of common occupations may suggest at-risk groups. Factories in LDCs often have minimal safety guidelines. Even when guidelines exist, they are frequently ignored. The net result is a high risk of personal injury and disfigurement. Accurate statistics regarding rates of personal injury from employment are difficult to locate. Brazil did not begin compiling statistics until 1969. In 1972, 18.1 percent of workers studied in Brazil had experienced an occupation-related injury [82]. Another study suggests that close to 50 percent of those injured were left with permanent incapacity [83]. The chance of being seri-

**Table 8.8
Factors which may increase the risks
and severity of work-related injuries**

Small shop size
Fatigue which increases the risk of accidents
  malnourished and stunted workers, sickness,
  long work hours in hostile environment (heat,
  humidity, poor lighting, etc.)
Environmental factors - heat, humidity, dust, toxins
Poorly maintained or outdated machinery - often lacking
  safety guards
Inadequate personal safety equipment
Inadequate preventive measures
Inadequate first aid or medical treatment available

ously injured was greater for workers in small shops than for workers in large factories [84]. This fact is particularly important because a significant proportion of shops in developing countries are very small. When a worker is permanently disabled, the worker may be fired and possibly given no compensation for the permanent loss of employability. Table 8.8 lists factors which may increase the risk of disability from occupational injuries.

Farmers may experience similar risk of personal injury. Almost no literature exists quantifying the rate and severity of disability. This is due in part to a lack of resources in the isolated rural regions. Another reason is the lack of a central monitoring department or agency. In addition, when a farmer is severely injured, the lack of transport facilities increases the risk of mortality and permanent disability. Personal experience in Liberia revealed numerous deaths caused by people being crushed under trees they were cutting down, and multiple injuries to extremities from cutlasses (Figure 8.11).

Occupational risks - poisonings. Both urban and rural inhabitants may run a risk of exposure to harmful man-made chemicals. WHO estimates that at least three million severe poisonings occur each year [85]. It has been estimated that up to 99 percent of these poisonings occur in less developed countries [86]. In developed countries, the main concern regarding chemical exposure is due to research that links long-term, low-level exposure to cancer and reproductive difficulties [87-91]. Workers in less developed countries run the risk of acute high-dose poisonings as well as the risk of long-term, low-level effects [92].

Figure 8.11

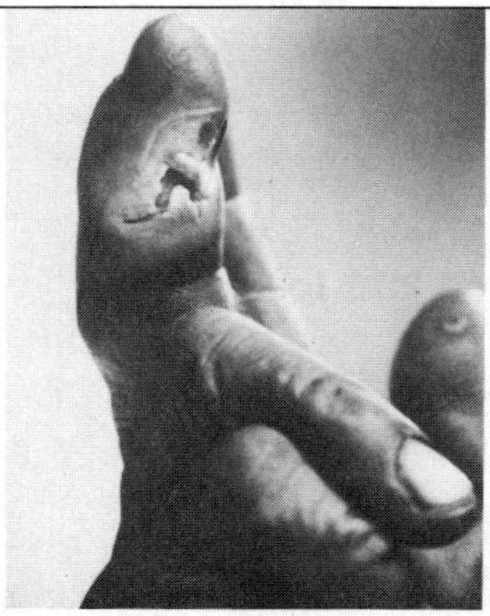

Farm-related injuries are very common. The finger shown became necrotic after a cutlass injury.

Both agricultural workers and pesticide manufacturing workers are at risk of acute pesticide poisoning. An average of 3 percent and 3.17 percent respectively become ill per year [93,94]. Organophosphate pesticides are the most common cause of acute poisonings. The risk of acute poisoning increases as the toxicity, dose and time of exposure increases. Most acute poisonings are felt to be avoidable. Ignorance regarding the toxicity of the pesticide appears to be the underlying cause of preventable exposures [95]. When people are educated regarding the health risks of inappropriate pesticide use, the risk of acute poisonings decreases [96].

Street children. Children living on the streets have numerous risks to their health. Although quantitative studies are few, it is believed that deaths due to violent crimes, drugs and auto accidents are on the increase for street children. In Brazil there are even reports of death squads which target street children. These at-risk children often make their living panhandling, selling small goods, prostitution or stealing. Street children will not have access to health care, immunizations or education. The chance of street children being identified for help is slim. With urbanization, the number of street children will increase.

Lifestyle. As is true in MDCs, lifestyle has a major impact on a person's health. The health risks of smoking are well documented. Nevertheless, smoking is on the rise among people in LDCs [97]. Urbanization and affluence may alter diet and activity levels causing an increase in diseases that commonly occur in Northern countries like heart disease and stroke.

Sexual promiscuity is acceptable in many societies. Because of the increased incidence of sexually transmitted diseases, including AIDS, this lifestyle practise places certain groups, such as prostitutes, at considerable personal risk. It is estimated that more than 85 percent of street prostitutes in Nairobi, Kenya are HIV positive [98]. J. Chin et al (1990) [99] estimate that up to 18 million people in the world will be HIV seropositive by the year 2000. For those people who have sexual relations with prostitutes or with multiple partners, the risk of AIDS is significant.

Summary. For each community, at-risk groups will vary. One can assume that women and children are at risk. Other groups with a high risk of illness can be identified by paying careful attention to locally prevalent causes of ill health. By first targeting at-risk groups, the greatest improvements can be realized given the limited resources available to most Third World communities.

C. Common and endemic diseases

Within each community certain diseases cause a disproportionate percentage of the morbidity and mortality. Diseases that are common, cause significant morbidity and are treatable must be identified. With this information, limited resources can then be used to treat the greatest number of people suffering from the most common illnesses.

Infectious diseases cause more morbidity and mortality for the inhabitants of developing countries than any other single disease group (Figure 8.12). Losing so many lives to treatable causes is sad. However, their treatable nature offers hope for improvement.

1. Disease prevalence and identification

Unless the health care worker is involved in direct patient care, many common illnesses may be overlooked. People often hide their illnesses and continue working even when quite sick. Attention to detail is necessary to recognize certain diseases. Mothers may dress their obviously malnourished children in frilly clothing. This directs the viewer's gaze to the clothing, and away from the child's wasted body. Long pants may hide tropical ulcers, the leopard skin of onchocerciasis, or the sores of dracunculiasis. Because of the social stigma attached to diseases like TB and leprosy, infected individuals will hide their symptoms. The ability to identify and diagnose ill people is enhanced if the fieldworker knows the locally prevalent diseases and is familiar with their typical presentation. This knowledge guides quick and accurate assessment.

The prevalence rates of selected diseases are available for most countries. This is an excellent starting point to direct the health care worker's investigation. Particular attention can be paid to disease entities known to exist in the community. However, it must be remembered that many common

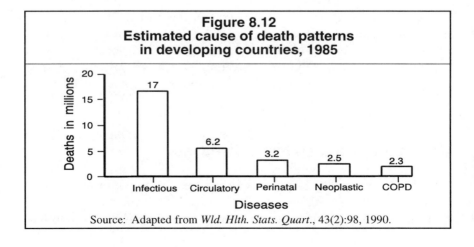

Figure 8.12
Estimated cause of death patterns
in developing countries, 1985

Source: Adapted from *Wld. Hlth. Stats. Quart.*, 43(2):98, 1990.

diseases may not appear in the published literature. An initial literature search will provide a foundation on which personal experience can build.

Western-trained health professionals who have little experience diagnosing diseases common to tropical regions may have great difficulty identifying maladies in indigenous people. Disease presentation is often different from the signs and symptoms described in textbooks. Malaria is an excellent example. Adult inhabitants of malarious regions may show none of the rigors, severe myalgias and cyclical fevers described in textbooks. Malaria often presents as a low grade fever, and the person feels mildly ill. For local people, malaria is like the viral flu with which Westerners are familiar.

The manifestations of certain diseases will also vary with the age of the affected person. For the young child, malaria can be the terrible illness described in tropical medicine textbooks. A small child will experience fevers, frequently cyclical, with a temperature rise up to 41 C, rigors, myalgias and impressive splenomegaly. If the child survives the infection, the body will create antibodies against the parasite. With each successive malaria infection the child survives, the immune response is strengthened. By adulthood, a malaria infection may resemble the flu more than the life-threatening illness it once was.

Schistosoma haematobium eggs are more likely to be found in the urine of a school-aged child than in an adult. Logic would suggest that older people have a longer exposure period and therefore are more likely to harbour the infection. What actually happens is that the older person develops a partial immunity to the infection, thereby decreasing the severity of infection and the number of eggs released in the urine.

Upon arrival at the project site, the health care worker should talk with a health care professional who has diagnostic experience of the endemic diseases, and who can describe their common presentations. This will assist the visiting health care worker to identify common diseases. It may actually be the only way to make correct diagnoses.

If any attempt is to be made at quantifying disease prevalence, criteria must be identified which constitute a specific diagnosis. For example, many different definitions for diarrhoea exist. The health worker needs to decide on one definition, and all survey members must use that definition. The Control of Diarrhoeal Diseases programme (CDD/WHO) has defined three or more loose stools in a 24-hour period as constituting diarrhoea

Table 8.9
Commonly-used diagnostic criteria for CHWs

Diagnosis	Symptoms and signs
Measles	Fever with red rash, red eyes, disappearing within a week
Poliomyelitis	Fever with paralysis
Trachoma	Chronic inflammation of the eyes, leading to shrinkage and turning-in of lids and blindness
Cholera	Sudden and severe watery diarrhoea with massive and rapid dehydration
Leprosy	Chronic hypopigmented skin lesions, loss of sensation, thickening of ear lobes, deformities of fingers, toes, and face
Tuberculosis	Cough for 4 weeks or longer, loss of weight, bloody sputum, low grade fever, night sweats
Trypanosomiasis	Fever, swollen glands in back of neck, lassitude, headache, sleepiness
Cutaneous leishmaniasis	Chronic, round, slowly healing ulcers, often on the face or exposed parts of body
Malaria	Fever, rigors, headache, body aches and inability to carry out normal daily activity. Splenomegaly present in children
Lymphatic filariasis	Fever, painful groin swellings, inflamed streaks in legs, elephantiasis, swollen genitals
Onchocerciasis	Itching of skin, nodules under skin, eye lesions, blindness
Schistosomiasis	Blood in urine of schoolchildren and teenagers
Ascaris	Roundworm expelled
Guinea worm	Painful legs, skin ulcers with worm protruding
Tapeworm infection	Segments expelled in faeces
Pneumonia	Fever and a rapid (>50bpm) respiratory rate
Diarrhoea	3 or more loose bowel movements in a 24-hour period
Diphtheria	Severe sore throat with difficulty breathing, fever and systemic toxicity
Pertussis	Upper respiratory infection with nonproductive cough and typical whoop
Tetanus	Tightness, spasticity, rigidity and paralysis of breathing
Neonatal tetanus	Failure to suck, weak cry, spasticity, seizures, and death in the first 3-28 days of life

Source: Adapted from *Manual of Epidemiology for District Health Management*, p. 50 and from R. B. Rothenberg, et al. [101]

[100]. If that is the diagnostic criteria chosen, then all people with three or more loose bowel movements in a 24-hour period must be classified as having diarrhoea.

The sophistication of the criteria chosen must match the abilities of the health workers. Resources must also be available to measure the selected criteria. If malaria is to be diagnosed only when the parasite is observed under the microscope, but no microscope exists and the health worker has never used a microscope, the data obtained from this survey will be inaccurate. Table 8.9 lists diagnostic criteria commonly used by local health workers. These symptoms and signs are obviously not the gold standards for diagnosis, but they are well suited for use by community health workers who need a functional definition.

These simple functional diagnostic criteria are quite useful for Western health care workers visiting developing countries. Many of the signs and symptoms are obvious. Health care workers should use every encounter with community members to further their understanding of the health problems common to the community. When the health worker meets a person on the road and stops to chat, the worker should note the person's physical characteristics. Deformities of limbs may suggest a prior polio infection. Open leg sores can suggest dracunculiasis or tropical ulcers. Depigmented patches of thickened skin could be leprosy. Emaciation can result from TB, AIDS or cancer. By careful observation during routine encounters, the astute health care worker can gain a wealth of information about common and endemic diseases.

A number of studies have used simple, easily identifiable signs or symptoms to obtain a crude estimate of disease prevalence in a community. The need for this simple tool exists because epidemiological information about the community is necessary to direct health interventions, but the resources to perform extensive experimental studies does not exist. What follows are a few examples of studies that used simple clinical findings or laboratory tests to identify disease prevalence of common maladies in developing countries.

2. Detection of onchocerciasis

Onchocerciasis is a significant public health concern in West Africa. It is best known as the cause of river blindness, but it has many other manifestations including lymphadenitis, dermatitis and onchocercomata. A number of diagnostic tests exist for the detection of onchocercal infection. The

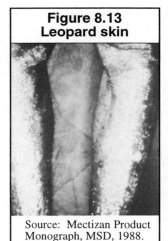

**Figure 8.13
Leopard skin**

Source: Mectizan Product Monograph, MSD, 1988.

gold standard is the demonstration of microfilaria in skin snips. Unfortunately, this method requires a sterile instrument to perform a skin biopsy, a microscope and a trained person to accurately examine the skin snip. Another method involves the identification of onchocercal skin nodules which represent the adult worm resting in the skin. This detection method involves examining the undressed patient to identify nodules which are found around the waist and upper legs. Barriers to the widespread use of this method include the need to undress, difficulty in locating nodules during light infections, and the possibility of confusing nodules with lymph nodes. The third diagnostic method involves the use of diethylcarbamazole (DEC) to induce the Mazotti reaction. The patient is given DEC and observed for two days to note any pruritis. At best there is inconvenience to the patient. However, the Mazotti reaction can sometimes be so severe that anaphylactic shock results. DEC use can also hasten the onset of onchocercal blindness.

L.D. Edungbola et al (1987) [102] have suggested using the presence of leopard skin (Ls) as a quick method of assessing the prevalence of onchocerciasis in a population. Leopard skin is a dermatological change associated with onchocercal infection that appears as multiple spots of depigmented skin (Figure 8.13). Although not every person with an onchocercal infection displays leopard skin, a significant number do, and the percentage appears to be somewhat constant. Therefore, Ls may not be a good screening tool for individual cases, but it can be used to gauge the prevalence of the disease in the population.

**Table 8.10
Prevalence of leopard skin (Ls) compared with the prevalence of skin microfilaria (mf)**

District	% with mf	% with Ls	Endemicity
1	9.7	0.8	Sporadic
2	48.6	8.9	Mesoendemic
3	62.4	9.8	Mesoendemic
4	28.5	4.6	Low
5	54.6	9.2	Mesoendemic

Source: Adapted from L. D. Edungbola, et al, (1987). *Int. J. Epidem.*, 16(4):591.

Leopard skin appears most frequently on the lower extremities. In warm climates legs are often exposed, thus enabling the casual observer to identify cases of onchocerciasis. Edungbola's study compared the microfilaria prevalence rates with the prevalence rates for leopard skin in the same populations. From this it was estimated that for a population with an Ls rate of less than one percent, the onchocercal infection was sporadic at best. An Ls frequency of between one and six percent corresponded to a hypoendemic state. Lastly, an Ls rate greater than six percent represented a meso- or hyper-endemic rate. Table 8.10 compares the prevalence of microfilaria to that of leopard skin. As can be seen, Ls occurs in only a small percentage of people harbouring microfilaria. It was found that the correlation coefficient comparing microfilaria prevalence and Ls prevalence was very good at 0.93. This implies a high degree of correlation, suggesting that Ls is a reliable indicator of onchocercal infection [102].

3. Night blindness - a screening tool for xerophthalmia

Recent research suggests that even mild Vitamin A deficiency significantly increases the morbidity and mortality rates in afflicted children [103]. When a child with Vitamin A deficiency develops another illness such as measles, the stress of the illness can further lower the Vitamin A level. This can precipitate xerophthalmia and can increase the child's chance of dying.

The most accurate method of assessing Vitamin A deficiency is by measurement of serum Vitamin A levels. This requires the drawing of blood, sophisticated laboratory equipment and the personnel to carry out the testing. Given these requirements, serum Vitamin A determination is an inappropriate screening tool in most developing communities.

A. Sommer et al [104] suggest using a history of night blindness as an accurate screening tool for identifying Vitamin A deficiency. Night blindness is the first symptom of clinically significant Vitamin A deficiency and may be followed by conjunctival xerosis and Bitot's spots (Figure 8.14). Because eye changes are a somewhat late sign and their identification requires a skilled examiner, a history of night blindness is commonly used as an indicator of early Vitamin A deficiency.

Dr. Sommer's survey team elicited a history of night blindness from a select population, and compared this information with the presence of xerotic changes and serum Vitamin A levels in the same population. Night blindness was considered present when the child's parent or guardian re-

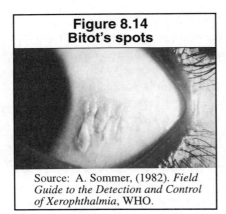

Figure 8.14
Bitot's spots

Source: A. Sommer, (1982). *Field Guide to the Detection and Control of Xerophthalmia*, WHO.

ported a strong history of the child's inability to locate food or toys in a poorly-lit room after dusk. In the population studied, night blindness was well known. A word for night blindness existed in the local language. It was noted that although a mother may not yet have recognized her child as being night blind, once she reached that conclusion through questioning, she was almost never wrong.

This study demonstrated that a strong history of night blindness was able to identify 84 percent of children with low serum Vitamin A level. The presence of Bitot's spots identified a lower percentage of children with a deficient Vitamin A level (41 percent). When a history of night blindness and/or the presence of Bitot's spots were combined, the two criteria served to identify all children with low serum Vitamin A levels. An interesting finding of this study was that children with low Vitamin A levels tended to live near one another. This suggests that when a number of children are identified as night blind in a neighborhood or area, all children in that area are at risk of being night blind. Therefore, it may be wise to treat all children in that area for Vitamin A deficiency.

This study demonstrates that night blindness is an excellent screening tool for Vitamin A deficiency. Given the relative ease and limited resources required to identify night blindness, this screening technique is applicable to many communities in developing countries. An added benefit is that the clustering effect of Vitamin A deficiency enables surveyors to identify many children at risk in a community using a small sample size. [85]

4. Haematuria and proteinuria as an indicator of schistosomiasis
Infection with *Schistosoma haematobium* is common and can lead to significant morbidity. Infection rates of 40 percent are common [105]. *Schistosoma*-related morbidity includes urinary bladder calcification, renal disease, hypertension and bacteriuria. Effective treatment options do exist, but limitations in field diagnosis have hindered treatment programmes. Urinary reagent dip sticks that test for haematuria and proteinuria are viable diagnostic tests.

WHO has recommended the use of Nuclepore urine filtration as the preferred method for *Schistosoma haematobium* diagnosis. The method is quite accurate, but its usefulness in developing countries is limited. Filter-based diagnosis requires filters, a vacuum apparatus, a microscope and a trained technician. These can be expensive. Some effort has been made to reduce the cost by reusing filters, but when washed incorrectly, the false positive rate increases [106].

Numerous authors have demonstrated that urinary reagent dip sticks which test for haematuria and proteinuria are accurate diagnostic tools [107,108]. When 2+ haematuria and proteinuria are present, reagent test strips can correctly diagnose 96 percent of infected cases. Higher levels of haematuria or proteinuria increase sensitivity to 100 percent. The level of haematuria directly correlates with the egg count [105]. The greater the haematuria, the larger the parasite burden. Reagent strip urinary haematuria is even more sensitive than parasitology for the diagnosis of light infections [108].

The field diagnosis of schistosomiasis using reagent strips requires the collection of urine. The urine is then tested by dipping the reagent strip in the urine and reading the haemoglobin and protein levels. If haematuria and proteinuria exist in the absence of other signs of urinary pathology (e.g. dysuria), a diagnosis of schistosomiasis can be made. Following treatment, the test can be used to measure efficacy.

Reagent strip measurement of urinary haematuria and proteinuria is an accurate method of diagnosing *Schistosoma haematobium* infection in the field. The method requires inexpensive reagent test strips and a minimally trained field worker. Given the low cost and simplicity, urinary reagent strip diagnosis of *Schistosoma* infection holds promise for use in low-income countries.

5. Estimating malaria prevalence

Malaria remains a major cause of morbidity and mortality. It is responsible for over one million deaths per year. Estimating the endemicity of malaria is helpful in understanding its impact on the health of a community. A greater improvement in a community's health will be realized if scarce resources are used to combat malaria in a hyperendemic area than in a hypoendemic area. Unfortunately, epidemiological assessment of malaria endemicity in rural areas of developing countries is not possible using modern measuring techniques due to the exorbitant costs and expertise involved in these methods. Estimating the prevalence of splenomegaly, a technique that has been used for years but has recently fallen out of favour, is a simple and inexpensive method that can provide useful information.

Detection of the malaria parasite in blood by light microscopy remains the method of choice for both clinical diagnosis and epidemiological measurement. Light microscopy has a number of drawbacks for use in rural village health posts. A light microscope is expensive, easily damaged, liable to need repairs requiring expensive imported parts, and requires a light source (either sunlight or mains current). Exhaustible supplies include microscope slides, immersion oil, stains and blood-drawing lancets. A greater obstacle to the general use of light microscopy is the need for a well-trained technician. Reading malaria smears requires a fair amount of expertise, is time-consuming and user fatigue results in decreased accuracy as the number of slides viewed per session increases. Epidemiological studies are beginning to use serum tests that measure antibody levels, but these tests are at present even less applicable than light microscopy.

Identifying the percentage of people in a community with splenomegaly is a simple and inexpensive method of estimating the prevalence of malaria. The method has been used successfully in a number of studies [79, 109]. Expensive equipment is not needed and the only requirement is a health care worker whose clinical skills include accurate assessment of spleen size. Considerable disagreement exists regarding the accuracy of the method [110,111]. When microscopy is possible, it should be used as the primary method and spleen size as an adjunct. For areas where microscopy is not possible, splenomegaly assessment is the method of choice.

In the tropics, the vast majority of enlarged spleens are due to infectious causes, particularly malaria. Schistosomiasis, kala-azar, typhoid and viral illnesses like hepatitis and measles also cause splenomegaly. Therefore, spleen rates may be less accurate in areas where other diseases like these are endemic. Protein energy malnutrition may skew spleen rates since some evidence suggests that undernutrition decreases the size of spleen enlargement. Finally, in communities where malaria is treated promptly, the spleen rate will be lower than expected. When evaluating a community for the rate of enlarged spleens these facts need to be noted and changes made in how the measured spleen rate is interpreted.

Acquired immunity changes the amount of splenic enlargement. With repeated malaria infections the spleen gradually increases in size. As malaria infections continue, a natural immunity develops which can decrease the amount of splenic enlargement. This decrease in spleen size often occurs by adulthood for people living in endemic regions. Because of this, it is best to evaluate children between two and nine years old when estimating the spleen rate. This decrease in spleen size with acquired immunity is also helpful when differentiating between areas where malaria is hyperendemic or epidemic. Adults in hyperendemic areas have smaller spleens than do adults who live in a non-endemic area and are experiencing a malaria epidemic. Children in hyperendemic areas have larger spleens than do children in epidemic areas although both spleen rates will be similar. Use of the average enlarged spleen index as described below attempts to quantify this relationship.

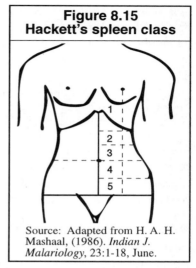

**Figure 8.15
Hackett's spleen class**

Source: Adapted from H. A. H. Mashaal, (1986). *Indian J. Malariology*, 23:1-18, June.

The examination of a patient for splenic enlargement is straightforward. The patient must be relaxed and in a supine position. The left side of the abdomen is palpated beginning at the pelvis and working superiorly up to the left costal border. Spleen size is then measured as the number of centimeters the spleen projects inferiorly below the costal margin along the left midclavicular line. For estimation of the average enlarged spleen index, a different measure is used. The degree of splenic enlargement is based upon landmarks on the patient. Splenic enlargement is broken down into five separate classes as defined by Hackett (Figure 8.15).

The most common reasons for missing an enlarged spleen include not starting the exam low enough in the abdomen, not recognizing a very soft spleen, and confusing massive liver enlargement with splenic enlargement. In young children the spleen may be enlarged into the pelvis. In a non-immune individual, the first few malaria infections result in a very boggy spleen that may be difficult to detect.

**Table 8.11
Malaria endemicity estimated from spleen rate**

Endemicity	Spleen rate (2-9 years)
Holoendemic	75-100%
Hyperendemic	50-75%
Mesoendemic	10-50%
Hypoendemic	0-10%

Source: F. J. Bennett, (1988). *Community Diagnosis and Health Action: A Manual for Tropical and Rural Area*. [112].

Spleen rate. The spleen rate is a simple percentage. The number of children aged two to nine who possess an enlarged spleen is divided by the total number of eligible children examined. This fraction is then multiplied by 100 to arrive at a percentage. Endemicity is then estimated from Table 8.11.

$$\text{Spleen rate} = \frac{\text{Number of children with splenomegaly}}{\text{Number of children examined}} \times 100$$

Average enlarged spleen index (AES). The average enlarged spleen index combined with the spleen rate can provide a more accurate estimate of the endemicity than either one taken separately. Whereas the spleen rate only considers a spleen as enlarged or not, the AES index takes into account the size of the spleen. This, as mentioned previously, can differentiate between hyperendemic areas and epidemic areas. Calculation of the average enlarged spleen index involves recording the Hackett's class of each individual. When the population has been surveyed, the number of individuals in each class is multiplied by the class number. This step is repeated for each class with the results from each multiplication added together. This sum is then divided by the number of people with enlarged spleens. When all enlarged spleens are class 1 the AES index equals 1.0. The greater the number of people with spleens in class 2 and above, the larger the AES index. In hyperendemic areas the average enlarged spleen index for children two to nine years old will be significantly above 1.0, while in non-endemic communities experiencing an epidemic, the AES will be closer to 1.0.

$$\text{AES} = \frac{\sum(\text{class number} \times \text{number of cases in class})}{\text{Number of cases with enlarged spleen}}$$

The spleen rate and the average enlarged spleen index are simple methods of estimating the endemicity of malaria in a community. They are best suited for areas where light microscopy is not possible. Careful application of these methods can provide information useful in directing health interventions.

Summary. In order to direct health interventions, information about common health problems must be available. Given the limited resources, health workers in developing countries must use innovative diagnostic methods to identify health problems correctly. The small number of methods presented meet these objectives. Further work must be devoted to develop similar methods.

References

1. UNICEF, (1981). Publicity Material, source unknown.
2. de Kadt E., Segall M., (1981). 'Health Needs and Health Services in Rural Ghana', *Soc. Sci. Med.,* 15A:421-517.
3. Wann T. T. H., Soifer S. J., (1974). 'Determinants of Physician Utilization: A Causal Analysis', *J. Health Soc. Behav.*, 15:100-108.
4. Wolinsky F. D., (1978). 'Assessing the Effects of Predisposing, Enabling and Illness-Morbidity Characteristics on Health Service Utilization', *J. Health Soc. Behav.*, 19:384-396.
5. Hershey J. C., Luft H. S., Giniaris J. M., (1975). 'Making Sense Out of Utilization Data', *Med. Care*, 13:838-854.
6. Fosu G. B., (1989). 'Access to Health Care in Urban Areas of Developing Societies', *J. Health Soc. Behav.*, 30:398-411.
7. Habib O. S., Vaughan J. P., (1986). 'The Determinants of Health Services Utilization in Southern Iraq: A Household Interview Survey', *Int. J. Epidem.*, 15(3)394-402.
8. Ghosh B. N., Mukherjee A. B., (1989). 'An Analysis of Health Services Coverage of a Primary Health Centre in West Bengal', *Ind. J. Pub. Hlth.*, 33(1):26-30, Jan-Mar.
9. Kadt E. D., Segall M. M., (1981). 'Health Needs and Health Services in Rural Ghana', *Soc. Sci. Med.*, 15A:417-427.
10. Okada L. M., Sparer G., (1976). 'Access to Usual Source of Care by Race and Income in Ten Urban Areas', *J. Comm. Health*, 1:163-174.
11. Cutts F. T., et al, (1990). 'Applications of Multiple Methods to Study the Immunization Programme in an Urban Area of Guinea', *Bull. WHO*, 68:769-776.
12. Ekunwe E. O., (1984). 'Expanding Immunization Coverage Through Improved Clinic Procedures', *World Health Forum*, 5:361-363.
13. Annis S., (1981). 'Physical Access and Utilization of Health Services in Rural Guatemala', *Soc. Sci. Med.*, 15D:515-523.
14. Balde M. D. and Bastert G., (1990). 'Decrease in Uterine Rupture in Conakry, Guinea by Improvements in Transfer Management', *Int. J. Gynecol. Obstet.*, 31:21-24.
15. Berardi J. C., Richard A., Djanhan Y., Papiernik E., (1989). 'Evaluation of the Benefit of Setting Up a Decentralized Obstetric-Surgical Structure in Order to Reduce Maternal Mortality and Transfers in Ivory Coast', *Int. J. Gynecol. Obstet.*, 29:13-17.
16. Munishi G. K., (1991). 'The Development of the Essential Drugs Program and Implications for Self-Reliance in Tanzania', *J. Clin. Epidemiol.*, 44(II):7S-14S.
17. WHO, (1985). *Handbook of Resolutions and Decisions of the World Health Assembly and Executive Board, Volume II, 1973-1984,* Geneva, World Health Organization:129.
18. Salako L. A., (1991). 'Drug supply in Nigeria', *J. of Clin. Epidem.*, 44 Suppl 2:15S-19S.
19. Waddington C., Panza A., (1991). 'Ten questions to ask about revolving drug funds', *Tropical Doctor*, Apr;21(2):50-3.

20. Royston E., Armstrong S., (1989). *Preventing Maternal Deaths*, WHO, Geneva, p. 137.
21. Billewicz W. Z., McGregor I. A., (1981). 'The Demography of Two West Africa (Gambian) Villages, 1951-1975', *J. of Biosoc. Science*, 13:219-240.
22. Eckholm E., Newland K., (1977). *Health: the family planning factor*. Washington, DC, Worldwatch Institute.
23. Jelliffe D. B., (1969). *Child Nutrition in Developing Countries, A Handbook for Fieldworkers*, USAID, Washington, DC.
24. Ferry B., Smith D., (1982). *World Fertility Study*, Available from TALC.
25. Morley D., Lovell H., (1990). *My Name is Today*, MacMillan Pub.,London, p.298
26. King J. and Ashworth A., (1987). 'Historical Review of the Changing Pattern of Infant Feeding in Developing Countries: The Case of Malaysia, the Caribbean, Nigeria and Zaire', *Soc. Sci. Med.*, 25(12):1307-1320.
27. *My Name is Today*, pp52-53.
28. Victora C. G., Barros F. C., Kirkwood B. R., Vaughan J. P., (1990). 'Pneumonia, Diarrhea, and Growth in the First 4 years of Life: a Longitudinal Study of 5914 Urban Brazilian Children', *Am. J. Clin. Nutr.*, 52:391-396.
29. WHO, (1990). *World Health Stats. Quarterly*, WHO, Geneva, Vol 43 (2),.
30. Choudhary S. R., Jayaswal O. N., (1989). 'Infant and Early Childhood Mortality in Urban Slums Under ICDS Scheme - A Prospective Study', *Indian Pediatrics*, 26:544-549, June.
31. *World Health Stats Quarterly*, (1990). Vol 42(2):98.
32. Morley D., (1969). 'Severe Measles in the Tropics', *Brit. Med. J.*, 1:297.
33. Chandra R. K., (1979). 'Nutritional Deficiency and Susceptibility to Infection', *Bull. WHO*, 57:167.
34. Kielmann A. A., McCord C., (1978). 'Weight for Age as an Index of Risk of Death in Children', *Lancet*, 1:860-862.
35. Chen L. C., Chowdhury A. K. M. A., Huffman S. A., (1980). 'Anthropometric Assessment of Energy-Protein Malnutrition and Subsequent Risk of Mortality Among Preschool Aged Children', *Am. J. Clin. Nutr.*, 33:1836-1845.
36. Martorell R., Yarbrough C., Yarbrough S., Klein R.E., (1980). 'The Impact of Ordinary Illnesses on the Dietary Intakes of Malnourished Children', *Am. J. Clin. Nutr.*, 33:345-350.
37. Hoyle B., Yunus M. D., Chen L. C., (1980). 'Breast-feeding and Food Intake Among Children with Acute Diarrheal Disease', *Am. J. Clin. Nutr.* 33:2365-2371.
38. Scrimshaw N. S., Taylor C. E., Gordon J. E., (1968). *Interactions of Nutrition and Infections*, WHO, Geneva, WHO: WHO Monograph no. 57.
39. Taddesse W. W., (1988). 'Immunoglobulins in Kwashiorkor', *East Afr. Med. J.*, 65(6):393-396, June.
40. Chandra R. K., (1975). 'Reduced Secretory Antibody Response to Live Attenuated Measles and Poliovirus Vaccines in Malnourished Children', *Br. Med. J.*, 2:583-585.

41. Munson D., Franco D., Arbeter A., Velez H., Vitale J. J., (1974). 'Serum Levels of Immunoglobulins, Cell-Mediated Immunity, and Phagocytosis in Protein-Calorie Malnutrition', *Am. J. Clin. Nutr.*, 27:625-628.
42. Schlesinger D., Stekel A., (19740. 'Impaired Cellular Immunity in Marasmic Infants', *Am. J. Clin. Nutr.*, 27:615-620.
43. Purtilo D. T., Riggs R. S., Evans R., Neafie R. C., (1976). 'Humoral Immunity of Parasitized, Malnourished Children', *Am. J. Trop. Med. Hyg.*, 25:229-232.
44. Koster F., Gaffar A., Jackson T. M., (1981). 'Recovery of Cellular Immune Competence During Treatment of Protein-Calorie Malnutrition', *Am. J. Clin. Nutr.*, 34:887-891.
45. Martorell R., Ho T. J., (1984). 'Malnutrition, Morbidity, and Mortality', In: Mosley WH, Chen LC, Eds. *Child Survival. Strategies for Research. Pop and Development Rev*, 10(suppl):49-68.
46. Black R. E., Brown K. H., Becker S., (1984). 'Malnutrition is a Determining Factor in Diarrhea Duration, but not Incidence, Among Young Children in a Longitudinal Study in Rural Bangladesh', *Am. J. Clin. Nutr.*, 39:87-94.
47. James J. W., (1972). 'Longitudinal Study of the Morbidity of Diarrheal and Respiratory Infections in Malnourished Children', *Am. J. Clin. Nutr.*, 25:690-694.
48. Trowbridge F. L., Newton L. H., Campbell C. C., (1981). 'Nutritional Status and Severity of Diarrhoea', *Lancet*, 1:1375(letter).
49. Mathur R., Reddy V., Naidu N., et al, (1985). 'Nutritional Status and Diarrheal Morbidity: A Longitudinal Study in Rural Indian Preschool Children', *Hum. Nutr. Clin. Nutr.*, 39C:447-454.
50. Black R. E., Brown K. H., Becker S., (1984). 'Effects of Diarrheas Associated with Specific Enteropathogens on the Growth of Children in Rural Bangladesh', *Pediatrics*, 73:799-805.
51. Mata L. J., Kromal R. A., Urrutia J. J., Garcia B., (1980). 'Effect of Infection on Food Intake Among Children with Acute Diarrheal Disease', *Am. J. Clin. Nutr.*, 33:2365-2371.
52. Martorell R., Yarbrough C., (1983). 'The Energy Cost of Diarrheal Diseases and Other Common Diseases in Children', In: Chen L. C., Scrimshaw N. S., Eds. *Diarrhea and Malnutrition. Interactions, Mechanisms, and Interventions.* New York: Plenum Press, 125-141.
53. Rowland M. G. M., Rowland S. G. J. G., Cole T. J., (1988). 'Impact of Infection on the Growth of Children from 0 to 2 years in an Urban West African Community', *Am. J. Clin. Nutr.*, 47:134-138.
54. Tupasi T. E., (1985). 'Nutrition and Acute Respiratory Infections', Eds. Douglas R. M. and Kerby-Eaton E., In: *Acute Respiratory Infections, Proceeding of an International Workshop, Sydney, August 1984*, University of Adelaide, Adelaide, 1985:68-71.
55. Escobar J. A., Dover A. S., Duenas A., et al, (1976). 'Etiology of Respiratory Infections in Children in Cali, Colombia', *Pediatrics*, 57:123-130.

56. Cohen N., et al, (1985). 'Prevalence and Determinants of Nutritional Blindness in Bangladeshi Children', *Wld. Hlth. Stats. Quart.*, 38:317-329.
57. Sommer A., Tarwotjo I., Hussaini G., Susanto D., (1983). 'Increased Mortality in Children with Mild Vitamin A Deficiency',
58. *Lancet*, ii:585-588.
    Sommer A., Katz J., Tarwotjo I., (1984). 'Increased risk of Respiratory Disease and Diarrhea in Children with Preexisting Mild Vitamin A Deficiency 1-3', *Am. J. Clin. Nutr.*, 40:1090-1095.
59. Jelliffe D. B., (1969).
60. Ross D. & Vaughan J. P., (1986). 'Health Interview Surveys in Developing Countries: A Methodological Review', *Stud. Fam. Plan.*;17(2):78-94, Mar-Apr.
61. UNICEF, *The State of the World's Children*, (1990). Oxford University Press, Oxford:23.
62. UNICEF, *The State of the World's Children*, (1990).
63. Mull J. D., Mull D. S., (1988). 'Mothers' Concepts of Childhood Diarrhea in Rural Pakistan: What ORT Program Planners Should Know', *Soc. Sci. Med.*, Vol 27(1):53-67.
64. Lerman S. J., Shepard D. S., Cash R. A., (1985). 'Treatment of Diarrhoea in Indonesian Children: What it Costs and Who Pays for it', *Lancet*, Sep 21.
65. Hazlett, D. T. G., et al, (1988). 'Viral Etiology and Epidemiology of Acute Respiratory Infections in Children in Nairobi, Kenya', *Am. J. Trop. Med. Hyg.*, 39(6):632-640.
66. Barclay, A. J. G., (1987). 'Vitamin A Supplements and Mortality Related to Measles: A Randomized Clinical Trial', *Br. Med. J.*, (294) 31 Jan:294-296
67. Pandey, M. R., et al., (1989). 'Indoor Air pollution in Developing Countries and Acute Respiratory Infection in Children', *Lancet*, 25 Feb:427-428.
68. Singhi S., Singhi P., (1987). 'Prevention of Acute Respiratory Infections', *Indian J. Pediatr.*, 54:161-170.
69. WHO, (1981). 'Clinical Management of Acute Respiratory Infections in Children: a WHO Memorandum', *Bull. WHO*, 59:707-16.
70. WHO, (1988). *Respiratory Infections in Children: Management in Small Hospitals. A Manual for Doctors*, World Health Organization, Geneva.
71. De Swardt R., Ijsselmuiden C. B., Edginton M. E., (1987). 'Vaccine Cold-Chain Status in the Elim Health Ward of Gazankulu', *S. Afr. Med. J.*, 72:334-336, 05 Sept.
72. Johnson S., Schoub B. D., McAnerney J. M., et al, (1984). 'Poliomyelitis Outbreak in South Africa, 1982. II. Laboratory and Vaccine Aspects', *Trans. Royal Soc. Trop. Med. Hyg.*, 78:26-31.
73. Carrasco R., Dinstrans R., Montaldo I., et al, (1982). 'Cold Chain and the Expanded Program on Immunization in Chile: an Evaluation Exercise', *Bull. PAHO*, 16(3):261-271.
74. UNICEF, *The State of the World's Children 1990*, p.18
75. Ahluwalia I. B., Helgerson S. D., Bia F. J., (1988). 'Immunization

coverage of children in a semi-urban village panchayat in Nepal, 1985', *J. Soc. Sci. & Med.*, 26(2):265-8.
76. Akesode F. A., (1982). 'Factors Affecting the Use of PHC Clinics for Children', *J. Epid. Com. H.*,36:310-314.
77. Alemu W., Woldeab M., Meche H., (1991). 'Factors Influencing Non-Attendance in the Immunization of Children in Three Selected Regions, Ethiopia, July 1988', *Ethiop. Med. J.*,29:49-55.
78. Molineaux L., Grammiccia G., (1980). *The Garki Project, Research on the Control of Malaria in the Sudan Savanna of West Africa*, Geneva, WHO, pp. 109-172.
79. Bradley A. K., Greenwood B. M., Greenwood A. M., et al, (1986). 'Bed-Nets (Mosquito-Nets) and Morbidity from Malaria', *Lancet*, 26 Jul:204-207.
80. Waswa, J. K., et al, (1988). 'The Nutritional Status of an Elderly Population in a Rural Area in Embu District, Kenya', *E. Afr. Med. J.*, Sep:578-587.
81. Bacley, A. C. (1982). 'Folacin, Iron Status and Hematological Findings in Predominantly Black Elderly Persons from Urban Low Income Households', *Am. J. Clin. Nutrit.*, 36:68.
82. Nogueira D. P., (1987). 'Prevention of Accidents and Injuries in Brazil', *Ergonomics*, 30(2):387-393.
83. Nogueira D. P., Gomes J. da R., Savaia N., (1981). 'Acidentes Graves do Trabalho na Capital do Estado de Sao Paulo', *Rev. Saude Publ.*,15:3-13.
84. Mendes R., (1975). *Importancia das Pequenas Empresas Industriais no Problema de Acidentes de Trabalho em Sao Paulo*, These, Faculdade de Saude Publica da Universidade de Sao Paulo, Sao.
85. World Health Organization/United Nations Environment Programme. *Public Health Impact of Pesticides Used in Agriculture.* Geneva, WHO.
86. Anon, (1985). 'Health Problems of Pesticide Usage in the Third World', *Br. J. Indust. Med.*, 42:505-506.
87. Ott M. G., Holder B., Gordon H., (1974). 'Respiratory Cancer and Occupational Exposure to Arsenicals', *Arch. Env. Health*, 29:250-255.
88. Mabuchi K., Lillienfeld A. M., Snell L. M., (1980). 'Cancer and Occupational Exposure to Arsenic; A Study of Pesticide Workers', *Preven. Med.*, 9:51-77.
89. Moody L., Halperin W. E., Fingerhut M. A., Landrigan P. J., (1984). 'The Chronic Health Effects of Occupational Exposure to Dioxin (Editorial Comment)', *Am. J. Indust. Med.*, 5:157-160.
90. Smith A. H., Fischer D. O., Pearce N., Chapman C. J., (1982). 'Congenital Defects and Miscarriages Among New Zealand 2,4,5-T Sprayers', *Arch. Environ. Health*, 37:197-200.
91. Townsend J. C., Brodner K. M., Van Peenen P. F., et al, (1982). 'Survey of Reproductive Events of Wives of Employees Exposed to Chlorinated Dioxins', *Am. J. Epidemiol.*, 115:695-713.
92. Shou-zhen Xue, (1987). 'Health Effects of Pesticides: A Review of Epidemiologic Research From the Perspective of Developing Nations', *Am. J. Indust. Med.*, 12:269-279.

93. Jeyaratnam J., et al, (1987). 'Survey of Acute Pesticide Poisoning Among Agricultural Workers in Four Asian Countries', *Bull. WHO*, 65(4):521-527.
94. Ou G. E., (1984). 'Nationwide Investigation of Occupational Poisonings by Lead, Benzene, Mercury, Organic Phosphorus Insecticides and Trinitrotoluene, with the Analytical Study of Their Etiology', *Chinese J. Indust. Hygiene Occup. Dis.*, 2:25-30.
95. Rosival L., (1985). 'Pesticides', *Scand. J. Work Environ. Health*, 11:189-197.
96. Jeyaratnam J., (1990). 'Acute Pesticide Poisoning: A Major Global Health Problem', *Wld. Hlth. Statist. Quart.*, 43:139-144.
97. Crofton J., (1990). 'Tobacco and the Third World', *Thorax*, 45:164-169.
98. Kreiss J., Kimball A. M., Holmes K. K., (1990). 'Global Patterns of HIV Infection', In: Holmes K. K., Collier A. C., Corey L., Handsfield H. H. Eds. *AIDS:Dx/Rx*. New York: McGraw-Hill.
99. Chin J., Sato P. A., Mann J. M., (1990). 'Projections of HIV Infections and AIDS Cases to the Year 2000', *Bull. WHO*, 68(1):1-11.
100. WHO/CDD/SER/80.2 Rev. 2, 1990.
101. Rothenberg R. B., et al, (1985). 'Observations on the Application of EPI Cluster Survey Methods for Estimating Disease Incidence', *Bull. WHO*, 63(1):93-99.
102. Edungbola L. D., et al, (1987). 'Leopard Skin as a Rapid Diagnostic Index for Estimating the Endemicity of African Onchocerciasis', *Int. J. Epidem.*, (16)4:590-594.
103. Barclay A. J. G., Foster A., Sommer A., (1987). 'Vitamin A Supplements and Mortality Related to Measles: A Randomised Clinical Trial', *Br. Med. J.*, 294:294-296, 31 Jan.
104. Sommer A., et al, (1980). 'History of Nightblindness: A Simple Tool for Xerophthalmia Screening', *Am. J. Clin. Nutrit.*, 33:887-891, Apr.
105. N'Goran K. E., et al, (1989). 'Screening for Urinary Schistosoma by Strips Reactive to Hematuria. Evaluation in Zones of Intermediate and Weak Endemicity in the Ivory Coast', *Bull. De La Soc. De Path. Exot. Et De Ses Fili.*, 82(2):236-242.
106. Mshinda M., et al, (1989). 'Field Diagnosis of Urinary Schistosomiasis by Multiple Use of Nuclepore Urine Filters', *J. Parasit.*;75(3):476-478, Jun.
107. Kassim O., (1989). 'Proteinuria and Haematuria as Predictors of Schistosomiasis in Children', *Ann. Trop. Paed.*, 3:156-160.
108. Taylor P., et al, (1990). 'Evaluation of the Reagent Strip Test for Hematuria in the Control of *Schistosoma hematobium* Infection in Schoolchildren', *Acta Tropica*, 47(2):91-100, Feb.
109. Moir J. S., Tulloch J. L., Vr Bova H., et al, (1985). 'The Role of Voluntary Village Aides in the Control of Malaria by Presumptive Treatment of Fever', *Papua New Guinea Med. J.*, 28:267-278.
110. Mashaal H. A. H., (1986). 'Splenomegaly in Malaria', *Indian J. Malarology*, 23:1-18, Jun.

111. De M. K., Chandra G., Chatterjee K. K., Hati A. K., (1990). 'Role of Splenomegaly in Diagnosis and Epidemiology of Malaria', *Indian J. Malarology*, 27:45-46, Mar.
112. Bennett F. J., Ed., (1979). *Community Diagnosis and Health Action: A Manual for Tropical and Rural Areas*, MacMillan Publ.:76.

Chapter 9

Rapid epidemiological assessment

Following the casual survey of a community, the health care worker may decide to study further the specific problems of the community. Health surveys are the most common tool used to measure health problems. The resources do not exist to sample every member of a community. Therefore, a number of techniques have been developed to select a segment of the population which is thought to represent the entire community. Rapid epidemiological assessment (REA) refers to sampling methods that attempt to accurately assess a population by using the fewest resources in the shortest time. These methods are suited to surveys in LDCs given the lack of resources and disease-reporting infrastructure. The strength of REA lies in its ability to elucidate causes of ill health quickly and inexpensively. This provides timely feedback to direct interventions.

Cluster sampling

Cluster sampling is a method of rapidly identifying representative members of a population. It is a general sampling technique that can be used to measure various disease prevalence rates. Cluster sampling was initially used by the expanded programme on immunization (EPI) to measure the vaccination coverage rates achieved by smallpox and measles immunization programmes [1]. Subsequent studies have shown the method useful in estimating disease incidence [2]. By simplifying the process of selecting subjects representative of the entire population, the cluster method has enabled epidemiological studies to be performed in isolated areas that would otherwise be too expensive to study.

Most survey investigations randomly select a small number of people from a population and then study only the selected individuals. This process requires that each member of the entire population be identified. Because the people under study are selected at random from the entire population, the results obtained are assumed to represent the results that would be obtained if the entire population had been included (within a certain confidence limit).

The random selection approach can be expensive in terms of time, money and personnel. For example, a rural area generally has a low population density. People are widely scattered in small villages. A rural population under study may contain 80 villages with the average number of village inhabitants being 100. A random sampling technique would first identify every member of the population, and then select individuals from almost every home in every village to attain the sample size dictated by statistical laws. This means the surveyor potentially must visit almost every home and every village to locate the individuals selected at random. This method requires a great deal of travelling. Many revisits may be required to locate people who were initially not found.

The cluster method simplifies the random selection process. There are many ways of performing a cluster sample. The modified two-stage method as used by the EPI will be discussed. The main assumption made in a cluster sample is that the variable under study is randomly distributed. Once the study population is defined, 30 or more sites (or clusters) are chosen. A random starting point is selected at each cluster site. From this starting point the first seven or more individuals contacted who meet the selection criteria are included in the study. This greatly simplifies the selection of the required number of subjects. Compared to the random sampling method, the cluster method requires identification of only the main sites (the 80 villages). The 30 sites from which the interviewees are obtained are randomly selected from the 80 villages. Once in the 30 selected villages, the interviewer selects the first seven people contacted who meet the selection criteria. There is no time spent tracking down specific people who were selected at random. This eases the process of selecting a statistically valid sub-population.

The number of clusters and the number of individuals in each cluster varies with a number of factors. If too few clusters are selected, the sample may not represent the entire population. If too many clusters are selected the method is not much faster than random sampling. The EPI has elected to use 30 clusters with at least seven subjects chosen from each cluster. This 30 x 7 structure was chosen because at least 192 individuals were needed to achieve statistical significance for their study. The total number of people in the sample population required to yield a statistically sound result is given by the standard formula for the variance of a binomial variable (Appendix 2, Equation 1). Once an estimate of sample size is calculated, the number of clusters can be selected for convenience (as long as there are at least 30 clusters if using the EPI method). The correct number of persons to choose from each cluster should be at least seven.

Immunization coverage and certain diseases tend to cluster. This can bias the results obtained from cluster sampling. The design effect is a way of describing how much the result obtained was influenced by disease clustering.

$$\text{Design effect} = \frac{\text{variance for cluster estimate}}{\text{variance for binomial estimate}}$$

When the design effect equals one, there is said to be no difference between using a cluster sampling technique and a completely random sampling technique. This suggests there was no clustering of disease prevalence by location. A design effect greater than one suggests clustering of the disease by location. Diseases that commonly begin at one focus and spread (e.g. epidemics) will result in a large design effect because both the disease and the sampling technique cluster. The use of the cluster-sampling technique for diseases which cluster may result in an overestimation of the prevalence of the disease.

In summary, the cluster-sampling technique is a useful means of selecting a representative sample when the factor under study does not cluster. Simplifying the process of sample selection is the significant strength of the method. Rothenberg et al (1985) [2] suggest that the cluster technique can also be used to compare disease trends over time. When used correctly, the cluster-sampling technique provides a simple and accurate means to assess health-related factors in economically disadvantaged countries [3,4].

Verbal autopsy

Many developing countries lack a vital registration system capable of recording all births, deaths and causes of death in the country. This is especially true in rural regions. People may die before reaching a health facility, or autopsy facilities may not be available. Without information about common causes of death, health care planners are ill-equipped to combat these problems. The verbal autopsy is a method of lay reporting which shows promise in providing information about the cause of death. It requires the construction of an algorithmic questionnaire which the deceased person's relatives answer. Based on their answers, an estimate of the cause of death is made. Although an actual autopsy may be the preferred method for identification of the cause of death, the verbal autopsy offers an alternative appropriate for use in less developed countries.

Implementation of the verbal autopsy requires the construction of a questionnaire. The questionnaire asks general demographic questions about the deceased. It then poses questions which narrow down the possible cause of death. These questions are algorithmic in nature. For example, if the main symptom identified by the family was a cough, the examiner would ask questions to identify the cause of the cough. Questions about the duration of cough, weight change, haemoptysis, associated fever, etc. would help to distinguish between tuberculosis, pneumonia or some other locally common cause of cough. If the main complaints were fever and rigors, the observer would use a different line of questioning.

The first step in constructing a verbal autopsy questionnaire is to identify locally common causes of death. This information can be obtained from published literature, local health workers and personal observation. Once the common diseases are catalogued, the second step involves the construction of a sign and symptom list for each illness. The list should be based on local disease presentation. Vernacular terms must be used to describe common conditions. The next and most difficult step requires construction of a diagnostic algorithm that will correctly identify the cause of death while excluding every other illness.

Once the questionnaire is designed, it must be translated into the local language. It is best to enlist the help of a bilingual community member as a translator. The community member verifies the questions' accuracy and clarity in the context of the local culture and language. It is helpful to have the questions posed to an indigenous person who then tells another interpreter what the question asked. This interpreter then translates that answer back into the language of the health care worker. If the original question and the question obtained through translation are different, there may be a problem with the original question.

After construction and translation, the questionnaire must be tested. Ideally, the questionnaire should be administered to family members who have had a relative die recently in a health facility and for whom a cause of death is known. The cause of death obtained from the verbal autopsy is compared with that of the hospital doctors. Once the questionnaire is constructed and tested, it is ready for use.

When a person in the study area dies, the closest friend or relative of the deceased is asked to participate in the verbal autopsy study. Care must be taken to observe all mourning rituals and customs. If the person agrees, an interviewer, preferably a literate community member, poses the questions. Because of recall bias, it is best to interview the relative within two to four weeks of the death. A longer period of time may diminish accuracy. The questionnaire should not take much longer than 30 minutes. Prolonged questioning can be intrusive in a person's life and may diminish local acceptance of the verbal autopsy tool. The completed questionnaire is then reviewed by a health care worker and a cause of death is assigned.

Pacque-Margolis et al (1990) found that in a select population, the verbal autopsy diagnosis agreed with the death certificate diagnosis in 80 percent of the cases [5]. They also found that the verbal autopsy questionnaire was cohort specific. A questionnaire constructed to diagnose adult deaths was less useful for accurate diagnosis of childhood deaths. This suggests that different verbal autopsy questionnaires must be constructed to diagnose all groups in the population.

The verbal autopsy is a viable tool for the estimation of cause of death for people in less developed countries. It is most useful where vital registration and autopsy facilities are inadequate. Constructing the questionnaire is difficult and must occur for each community and each cohort group. Once the questionnaire is constructed, the input of time and resources is minimal. In addition to estimating the prevalence of leading causes of death, the method holds promise for tracking changes in the cause of death over time [5].

Estimating maternal mortality by the sisterhood method

Maternal mortality is a significant health problem. An estimated 500 000 pregnancy-related deaths occur annually. The actual number of maternal deaths per year is unknown because of inadequate vital registration. Community-based surveys of maternal mortality are also scant. Given an average maternal mortality ratio (MMR) of 50 - 1 000 per 100 000 live births, the size of the population that must be followed is huge. A community-based survey method is too costly for most developing nations. The sisterhood method of estimating maternal mortality is meant to address this shortcoming.

Wendy Graham et al (1989) described the sisterhood method as a technique that

> uses the proportions of adult sisters dying during pregnancy, childbirth, or the puerperium reported by adults during a census or survey, to derive a variety of indicators of maternal mortality [6].

A main attraction of this method is that by interviewing just one sibling, maternal mortality information is obtained for all female siblings of reproductive age in the family. Given the large family size prevalent in traditional societies, interviewing one family member can provide information on many women. This means that a statistically significant sample size can be achieved with much less effort. Even when the time between maternal death and interview is long, it is felt that a childbirth-related death is quite memorable. Although the date of death and the age at death may be forgotten, the death itself will not be forgotten. Recall bias is therefore less a factor. Finally, the sibling report is felt to be accurate because many siblings keep in touch even after leaving the nuclear family.

The reason the sisterhood method of estimating maternal mortality is possible is because a proportional relationship exists between the proportion of sisters to have died as reported by a sibling of a certain age, and the probability of these women dying by a certain age. This relationship can be used to estimate a woman's lifetime risk of maternal death. Appendix 2, Equation 2, discusses this relationship more fully.

The sisterhood method requires asking only five questions.

1. The age of the respondent?
2. How many sisters (born to the same mother) have you ever had who were ever married or who have reached the age of marriage (including those who are now dead)?
3. How many of these ever-married sisters are alive now?
4. How many of these ever-married sisters are dead?
5. How many of these dead sisters died while they were pregnant, or during childbirth, or during the six weeks after the end of pregnancy?

The age of the respondent is important because siblings' ages cluster. Younger respondents are more likely to have sisters who have not yet entered the childbearing period and therefore are not yet at risk of maternal mortality. The opposite holds true when the respondent is elderly. Because personal age may not be known, a calendar of locally significant events may need to be constructed so a rough idea of the respondent's age can be estimated.

Question two tries to define the population at risk of maternal death. A woman must have entered menarche and must be sexually active to be exposed to the chance of maternal death. Menarche occurs at different ages for different women, but is generally taken to be age 15. In some societies, sexual activity can only occur within the confines of marriage. In other societies, sexual activity may be permissible any time after menarche. Because of this, question two must be worded in a culturally appropriate way to identify women of reproductive age who are sexually active.

Questions three and four are designed as a cross check for the answer to question two. They identify the total number of the respondent's sisters. Question five identifies the number of sisters who died as a result of pregnancy. The wording of question five is based upon the international classification of disease (ICD-9) definition of a maternal death. For a death to be recorded as a maternal death, the woman must have died of a pregnancy-related cause any time during the pregnancy, during childbirth or within 42 days postpartum. If the death occurred from a non-pregnancy-related cause such as an auto accident or occurred outside the time frame defined, the death is not considered a maternal death. Since many traditional societies are not chronologically-oriented, a locally common unit of measure for 42 days must be identified.

Once the questions are in a culturally acceptable form and have been tested for accuracy, interviewers can question all male and female adults in the community. Interviewers should be literate members of the community who have been trained in use of the questionnaire. The gender of the respondent should be recorded on the questionnaire for later use. In some societies, men have little knowledge of women-related issues. If this is true and the sample population is large enough, male-female respondent results should be analyzed separately. Since the calculation of lifetime risk of maternal mortality is based on a proportion, it is acceptable and desirable to interview all siblings [7].

Based on the information obtained from the survey, an estimate of the lifetime risk of maternal death can be calculated.

$$\text{Lifetime risk of maternal death} = \frac{\text{Number of maternal deaths reported}}{\text{Number of ever-married sisters} \times \text{adjustment factor}}$$

From Dr Graham's example the lifetime risk of maternal death equals 0.0584. Dividing 1 by the lifetime risk of maternal death (0.0584) provides an estimate of a woman's lifetime risk of dying in childbirth. Therefore, for the example given, a woman has a 1 in 17 chance of dying in childbirth for the study population. This 1 in 17 chance can be converted to the more commonly used value of the maternal mortality ratio by the following equation:

$$\text{MMR} = \left(1 - (\text{Probability of Survival})^{(1/\text{TFR})}\right) \times 100{,}000$$

where:
> Probability of survival = 1 - lifetime risk of maternal death, and
> TFR = total fertility rate.

The sisterhood method of estimating maternal mortality is an indirect survey method of estimating the MMR. It has successfully addressed a major stumbling block in the estimation of maternal mortality; namely, the huge sample population required by direct survey techniques to estimate the MMR accurately. The questionnaire is simple, and the entire interview process brief. The calculations are also quite simple, and can be performed on a hand calculator. When used in an epidemiologically-sound fashion and in an appropriate population, the sisterhood method provides a simple tool for estimating maternal mortality. This inexpensive and easy method holds promise in guiding health care planners in health interventions.

Questionnaires aimed at key informants

Estimating disease prevalence remains a difficult and costly undertaking. Using accepted epidemiological tools, such as light microscopy for malaria or urine filtration for schistosomiasis, may consume a sizeable percent of a district health unit's budget. This can leave inadequate funds to identify other significant health problems, and limited money to combat the identified problems. Health workers are beginning to acknowledge that community members have an excellent awareness of disease symptomatology for many of the common diseases they experience [8]. C. Lengeler et al have used this fact to identify areas of high disease prevalence by questioning key informants and community members [9-11].

By asking headteachers and school children to complete simple questionnaires, Lengeler et al identified schools where a high percentage of the children were infected by *Schistosoma haematobium*. The method is quite simple and involves creating a simple questionnaire that is culturally appropriate; distributing the questionnaire through pre-existing delivery systems; having the key informants (i.e. headteachers) complete their questionnaire and interview their students regarding symptom and disease occurrence; and cross validation of the results reported by the key informants using a subset of the entire study population. Although the method is qualitative in nature, it is very good at excluding low-risk populations, and at identifying areas that need further study. The method is extremely cost-effective. Lengeler's studies cost 24-26 times less than a similar study using the accepted method of urine filtration. As with most epidemiological methods, it is useful for identifying populations at risk of illness. However, it cannot be used as a clinical tool to identify ill patients. For schistosomiasis, urine dipstick testing can identify individual patients accurately and inexpensively. Lengeler et al have shown the usefulness of questioning key informants to identify areas with high *Schistosoma* prevalence. Further studies must be performed to estimate the method's usefulness for identifying other endemic illnesses.

For the method to be useful, a number of criteria must be met. The disease under study must have easily identifiable symptoms that community members recognize. The disease under study must be considered important by people in the community. Health workers and community members may disagree on the importance of certain diseases, but if community members do not perceive the disease to be important, they are less likely to identify its symptoms. A list of common health problems must either be available or must be created before the questionnaire can be constructed. Finally, an intact social structure such as a school system or political system must exist for the identification of key informants and the distribution of questionnaires. To avoid significant bias, the selected social structure must penetrate to all members of the study population. For example, if a school system is the selected social structure, but school attendance is low, a significant, and often high-risk, proportion of the population will not be screened.

Questionnaire creation and completion. As outlined by Lengeler et al, the key informant's questionnaire consisted of six questions and the student's questionnaire of two. An important point to note is that the key informants should be told the questionnaire is a general health survey and is not targeted at one disease. Disclosing which disease is under study can result in erroneous answers. Given this fact, the questionnaire is constructed as a general health survey asking questions about many topics. Question one of the Lengeler study presented a list of diseases that were thought to be common in children and asked the key informants to rank the diseases in importance. Question two presented a list of common signs and symptoms in children and asked the key informant to rank these from most to least prevalent. Question three asked the key informants to create their own list of prevalent diseases that should be a priority for control. Question four provided a list of village problems that the key informants were to rank. Question five and six dealt with health facilities and water supplies.

The student questionnaire asked whether the student had had any of the listed signs or symptoms in the past month, and whether the student had had any of the listed diseases in the past month. These questions were posed to the student in private by the student's headteacher.

As with the construction of any questionnaire, these questionnaires must be based on locally prevalent terminology, and must be written in the local language. The questionnaires must be tested on a small group of people who mirror the general characteristics of population members. Lengeler found that the questionnaires were well received with close to 100 percent return and completion rates.

Cross validation. Cross validation may be the most expensive part of this method. When baseline biochemical data are not available for the study population, a subset of the population must be tested using some biochemical method. This sub-sample data is then used to determine which questions can differentiate between areas of low and high prevalence. Lengeler et al have used urine filtration and urine dipstick biochemical measures. They compared egg prevalence rate or level of haematuria prevalence rate to individual questions from the questionnaire. From this comparison they maximized sensitivity and specificity by selecting a specific question and a specific rank level. For example, the sensitivity and specificity of identifying high-risk schools was maximized if the key informant's response to question three had a rank of four or less (schistosomiasis control was listed by the headteachers as one of the top four priority interventions). Therefore in all schools where the headteachers felt that schistosomiasis control was of low priority, the risk of children in that school experiencing significant schistosoma morbidity was low. In schools where headteachers ranked schistosomiasis control as a priority, the risk of children having significant *Schistosoma* morbidity was high. In other words, teachers' perceptions that schistosomiasis was a significant health problem were quite accurate.

One significant exception to this rule occurred in a school where a schistosomiasis control programme had been active. In spite of the control effort, the egg prevalence rate in the community remained high. The fact that the control programme had been in the community seemed to change people's perception regarding schistosomiasis as a problem. Although the egg prevalence rate was high, people felt that schistosomiasis was no longer a problem. Further work needs to be done on this relationship. If this effect is common, the questioning of key informants may be useful only for initial studies.

Questionnaires aimed at key informants hold promise as an inexpensive and reliable method to identify high- and low-risk populations for selected diseases. The method's strengths include: non-invasive nature, low cost, ability to obtain useful information rapidly from a large population, and limited burden on an already over-stressed health care system. The method's shortcomings include: the need for an intact social structure to distribute the questionnaire and perform the testing, the limited number of diseases that can be studied, the requirement that community members must perceive the disease as important, and the way health interventions change community members' perception of a disease's importance. Many of these shortcomings may become less important as the method is refined.

REA summary

Rapid epidemiological assessment techniques extend the collection of epidemiological information to the poorest and most isolated regions by decreasing the amount of time and resources required to obtain statistically valid results. This should not result in losing sight of the purpose of performing community assessment. The primary objective of assessment is to produce useful information to guide health care workers and planners in combating the identified problems. Community assessment is a tool. It is not an end in itself. The desire to assess a community should arise from the desire to improve the health and well-being of the community and its members. The health care worker's initial exposure to the community should help him or her identify possible problems. A health survey further elucidates the identified problems and guides interventions. By remembering these points, more time will be spent intervening and less time spent repeating similar studies.

Cluster sampling, verbal autopsy, the sisterhood method and questioning key informants are four examples of rapid epidemiological assessment techniques. Many other REA techniques are available or are being developed. The article by Gordon Smith [12] provides a starting point for readers interested in identifying other rapid assessment techniques.

Rapid epidemiological assessment techniques ease the process of community assessment, but do not remove the need for sound epidemiological rigour. A poorly done REA study is as useless as a poorly done traditional assessment. Attention must be paid to the design and execution of the study. Appendix three lists important guidelines which should be followed during any epidemiological survey.

References

1. Henderson R. H., et al, (1973). 'Assessment of Vaccination coverage, vaccination scar rates, and smallpox scarring in five areas of West Africa', *Bull. WHO*:48:183-194.
2. Rothenberg R. B., et al, (1985). 'Observation on the application of EPI cluster survey methods for estimating disease incidence', *Bull. WHO*:63(1):93-99.
3. Lemeshow S., (1988). 'Sampling Techniques for Evaluating Health Parameters in Developing Countries', BOSTID, National Academy Press, Washington, DC.
4. Henderson R. H., Sundaresan T., (1982). 'Cluster sampling to assess immunization coverage: a review of experience with a simplified sampling method', *Bull. WHO*:60(2):253-260.
5. Pacque-Margolis S., et al, (1990). 'Application of the verbal autopsy during a clinical trial', *Soc. Sci. Med.*, Vol 31, No. 5:585-591.
6. Wendy Graham, William Brass, Robert W. Snow, (1989). 'Estimating Maternal Mortality: The Sisterhood Method', *Stud. Fam. Plan.*:20(3):125-135.
7. Trussell J., Rodriguez G, (1990). 'A Note on the Sisterhood Estimator of Maternal Mortality', *Stud. Fam. Plan.*:21(6):344-346, Nov/Dec.
8. Jackson L. C., (1985). 'Malaria in Liberian Children and Mothers: Biocultural Perceptions of Illness vs. Clinical Evidence of Disease', *Soc. Sci. Med.*, 20(12):1281-1287.
9. Lengeler C., de Savigny D., Mshinda H., et al, (1991). 'Community-Based Questionnaires and Health Statistics as Tools for the Cost-Efficient Identification of Communities at Risk of Urinary Schistosomiasis', *Int. J. Epidemiol.*, 20(3):796-807.
10. Lengeler C., Kilima P., Mshinda H., et al, (1991). 'Rapid, Low-Cost, Two-Step Method to Screen for Urinary Schistosomiasis at the District Level: The Kilosa Experience', *Bull. WHO*, 69(2):179-189.
11. Lengeler C., Mshinda H., de Savigny D., et al, (1991). 'The Value of Questionnaires Aimed at Key Informants, and Distributed Through an Existing Administrative System, for Rapid and Cost-Effective Health Assessment', *Wrld. Hlth. Stats. Quart.*, 44:150-159.
12. Smith G.(1989). 'Development of Rapid Epidemiologic Assessment Methods to Evaluate Health Status and Delivery of Health Services',*Int. J. Epidem.:*18(suppl 2):S2-S15.

Appendix
International agricultural research centres

Centre	Programme areas
Centro International de Agricultura Tropical (CIAT) Apartado Aereo 6713 Cali, Colombia	a. Dry beans b. Cassava c. Tropical pasture d. Rice
Centro International de Mejoramiento de Maiz y Trigo (CIMMYT) Londres 40 Mexico, D.F., Mexico	a. Maize b. Wheat c. Economics
International Center for Agriculture Research in the Dry Areas (ICARDA) P.O. Box 114/5055 Beirut, Lebanon	a. Cereals (wheat, barley, tritacale) b. Legumes (lentils, faba, chick peas) c. Forages
International Crops Research Institute for the Semi-Arid Tropics (ICRISAT) Patancheru P.O. Andhra Pradesh 502324 India	a. Sorghum b. Pearl millet c. Pigeon peas d. Chick peas e. Groundnuts f. Farming systems
International Institute of Tropical Agriculture (IITA) P.O. Box 5320 Ibadan, Nigeria	a. Root and tuber crops b. Grain legumes (cowpeas, soybeans) c. Farming systems
International Livestock Center for Africa (ILCA) P.O. Box 5689 Addis Ababa, Ethiopia	a. Livestock production and marketing systems
International Rice Research Institute (IRRI) Manila, Philippines	a. Rice production, genetic evaluation and utilization b. Cropping systems c. Small-scale farm machinery
West African Rice Development Association (WARDA) E.J. Roye Memorial Building P.O. Box 1019 Monrovia, Liberia	a. Rice production, processing and marketing b. Seed multiplication
Asian Vegetable Research and Development Center (AVRDC) P.O. Box 42 Shanhua, Tainan 741 Taiwan, Republic of China	a. Tomatoes b. Chinese cabbage c. Sweet potatoes d. Mung beans e. Soybeans

Adapted from: E. B. Oyer, (1984). 'Agricultural Research and Technology Transfer for Food Production: What Strategies Are Appropriate?', *World Food Issues*, Second Ed., Cornell University, pp. 65-71.

REA equations

Binomial equation

Equation 1:

$$n = ((z \times z) \times p \times q) / (d \times d)$$

where:
n = number of persons required in the sample
d = the precision of the result desired
z = the confidence limits of the survey results
p = the proportion of people who have the factor under study
    This is a best-guess estimate
q = 1 - p

Sisterhood equation

The reason the sisterhood method of estimating maternal mortality is possible is because a proportional relationship exists between the (proportion of sisters to die as reported by a sibling of age u = psi(u)) and (the probability of dying by age u = q(u)).

Equation 2:

$$psi(u) \sim q(u)$$

By applying an adjustment factor, 'A', to the left side of the equation

$$A \times psi(u) \sim q(u)$$

an estimate can be made of the life time risk for maternal death. 'A' must take into account the age of the respondent. Because siblings' ages cluster, it is common for a young respondent to have siblings who are also young, and have either recently entered the childbearing years, or have yet to enter them. This means the siblings of a young respondent are less likely to have died, because their exposure to the risks of childbirth is small. For the respondent who is old (50+), most of that person's siblings will have already completed their childbearing years so the total number of siblings who died in childbirth will be known. This means the adjustment factor, 'A', varies with the age of the respondent. Dr. Graham lumped respondents' ages in five year groups and calculated the 'A' for each age group. For more information on the derivation of this relationship and examples of calculations, the reader is referred to W. Graham et al, (1989) [Chapter 9, Reference 6].

Health survey guidelines

1) The primary objective of assessment is to improve the health of the community and its members.
2) Survey results must be communicated widely. In particular, the results must be shared in an understandable way with the community that was measured.
3) The objectives of the survey should be clearly defined in quantitative terms and the study design should address the objectives.
4) Multi-stage random sampling techniques like the cluster method are the most efficient way of selecting the sample population. The study design should limit the need to locate specific community members.
5) Interviewers should be chosen from the study area and should share common cultural features like language and religion with community members.
6) For interview surveys, interviewers should not be medically trained.
7) Proxy responding to interview questions should be avoided except for the survey of young children.
8) Unless the event being measured is salient (e.g. death of sibling), a recall period of two to four weeks is best.
9) An annual rate cannot be estimated unless a survey is continued for an entire calendar year. This is because many phenomena exhibit a seasonal variation.
10) Because of this seasonal variation, repeat surveys should be carried out at the same time of year and surveys that were performed during different seasons should only be compared with extreme caution.
11) For questionnaires, the order of the questions matters.
12) Tracer conditions should be used to allow standardization between surveys.
13) Some measure of illness severity should be performed.
14) Surveys which attempt to gauge health facility use rates should not ignore the use of traditional healers and other health personnel recognised as such by the community.
15) All questionnaires should by tested on people with cultural characteristics similar to the sample population.
16) Internal consistency checks of completed questionnaires should be performed daily to provide feedback to interviewers on problems which need correction.

The above points were taken from: David A. Ross & J. Patrick Vaughan, (1986). 'Health Interview Surveys in Developing Countries: A Methodological Review', *Stud. Fam. Plan.*, 17(2):78-94.

Sources for published materials pertaining to international health

Blackwell
50 Broad Street
Oxford OX1 3BQ, UK   Tel: (0865) 792792

Information Collection and Exchange (ICE)
Peace Corps

Intermediate Technology Publications
103-105 Southampton Row
London, WC1B 4HH, UK   Tel: 071-436 9761

Intermediate Technology Development Group of North America, Inc.
Publications Office
P.O. Box 337
Croton-on-Hudson, NY 10520, U.S.A.

International Children's Centre
Chateau de Longchamp
75016 Paris, France   Tel: 1 45 20 79 92

Oxford University Press
2001 Evans Road
Cary, NC 27513, U.S.A.

Teaching Aids at Low Cost (TALC)
P.O. Box 49, St. Albans
Herts. AL1 4AX, UK Tel: (0)727 53869

Third Party Publishing Company
P.O. Box 13306, Montclair Station
Oakland, CA 94661-0306, U.S.A.   Tel: 415/339-2323

World Health Organization (Subscriptions)
Distribution and Sales
1211 Geneva 27, Switzerland

World Health Organization (Books)
WHO Publications Center USA
49 Sheridan Ave.
Albany, NY 12210, U.S.A.

World Neighbors
5116 North Portland Avenue
Oklahoma City, OK 73112, U.S.A.   Tel: (405)946-3333

Index

A

abruptio placenta   36
access   6, 8, 14, 16, 26, 75, 79-81, 83, 84, 87, 89-91, 100, 103
accidents   14, 18, 20, 93, 103
acute respiratory infection;   *see* ARI
adobe   66
AES (average enlarged spleen)   113, 114
affluence   103
affordability   84
Africa   18, 27, 43, 57, 89, 90, 107
agriculture 1, 10, 49, 51, 60
AIDS   18, 103, 107
algae   57
Alma Ata   1
anaemia   35, 36
anaemic   35, 36, 100
anaphylactic shock   108
animist   8, 84
Anopheles 30, 99
anthropologist   82
anthropology   11
antibiotics   85, 97
ARI (acute respiratory infection) 3, 94-97
assessment   1-8, 10, 11, 13, 44, 60, 63, 75, 78, 79, 87, 95, 104, 111, 112, 123, 133, 134
Aswan dam   31
at-risk 6, 79, 88, 100, 101, 103
autopsy, verbal   125-127, 133
average enlarged spleen; *see* AES

B

bacteria   25, 27, 42, 56, 96
bacteriuria 110
bank   50, 75
barriers   19, 20, 27, 79, 81-83, 100, 108
bathe   29
bednets   99
bias   5, 6, 10, 82, 124, 131
    recall   126, 128
bicycle   20, 68
bilharziasis   101;   *see also* schistosomiasis
binomial   124, 136
biopsy   108
birds   25, 59
birth attendant   64, 89, 91
birth control   84, 89

birth interval   15, 16
birthweight   36, 37, 94, 97, 98
births   16, 88, 92, 125, 127
Bitot's spots   109, 110
black fly   30
blacksmith   19, 63
blindness   30, 101, 107-110
blood   109
books   60, 76
bottle-feeding   17, 37, 38, 97
bowl   39
breast-feeding   17, 37, 44, 63, 90, 97

C

caag   53, 54
calcification   110
caloric   28, 35, 37, 38, 41, 53, 68, 94
cancer   40, 102, 107
car   67, 68
carpenters   63
carts   68
cash cropping   49
cassava   38, 52
CDD   (control of diarroeal diseases)   105
cement   26, 66
centrifuge   70
cephalopelvic disproportion; *see* CPD
cercaria   29;   *see also* schistosomiasis
cereal   52, 56
cheese   42
chemicals   21, 26, 55, 58, 102
childbearing   16, 88, 89, 91, 128
childbirth   16, 17, 128, 129
child labour   20
children   13, 15-17, 20, 21, 28, 29, 36, 38, 39, 41, 42, 56, 63, 79, 87-100, 104, 109, 110, 112-114, 130-132
   street   103
chlamydia   18
chloroquine   99, 100
Christian   84
CHW (community health worker)   6, 64, 84, 85, 106, 107
circumference, arm   94, 95
clay   66
clinics   6, 64, 84, 85, 107
cluster sampling   123-125, 133
coal   58, 67
cold chain   97, 98
community
   assessment   1-3, 7, 8, 10, 11, 60, 63, 75, 78, 79, 133, 134

definition   2
evaluation   3
health worker;   *see* CHW
composting   57
contraception   90
contraceptive   89-91
cook   39, 40-42
cookstoves   40, 56, 65
copper   55
corn   38
cost   6, 15, 20, 26, 51, 64-68, 70, 72, 75, 76, 83, 85-87, 96, 111, 131, 133
cough   126
country devil   8
coverage   80, 82, 83, 87, 97, 98, 123, 124
cow peas   56
CPD (cephalopelvic disproportion)   35
craftspeople   63, 64, 75
credit   18, 87
crimes   14, 103
crops   28, 51-57, 59
cross validation   130, 132
cultivation   49, 53

D

death   13, 35, 36, 67, 73, 92-98, 100, 102, 103, 111, 125-129
   maternal   36, 128, 129, 130
debt   50, 73, 87
DEC (diethylcarbamazole)   108
defecate   28, 29
deficiency
   iodine   36
   iron   36
   potassium   55
   Vitamin A   94, 109, 110;   *see also* night blindness, xerophthalmia
deforestation   40, 41, 52
dehulled   59
dehydration   95-97
demographics   13, 18-21, 80
density, population   13-15, 18, 83, 124
dermatitis   107
desertification   41, 52, 57
design effect   124-125
diagnostic   84, 85, 105, 107, 108, 110, 111, 122, 126
diarrhoea   1, 27, 94-97, 105, 107
dishes   27
disrespect   83
distance   20, 81, 83
distribution   13, 39, 94, 100, 131

donkey   70
drugs   85-87, 103;   *see also* medicine
drug store   83, 84
drying   42, 60
dung   56

E

EC (european community)   9, 75
economic status   16, 19, 20
education   9, 16, 19, 20, 27, 64, 76, 87, 90, 91, 96, 98, 103
educational level   16, 19, 21, 81, 84, 90, 91
eggs   43, 105, 111, 132
Egypt   31
elderly   100, 128
electricians   63
electrical power   85
electricity   70-72
embassies   74
endemic   79, 81, 82, 99, 103, 105, 107, 112, 131
energy   25, 28, 38, 53, 68-72
EPI (expanded programme on immunization)   123, 124
erosion   57, 58
essential medicines   85-87
excreta   28, 29
expanded programme on immunization;   *see* EPI

F

facilities   7, 26, 81, 84, 85, 102, 125, 127
   health   14, 19, 67, 80, 83, 84, 87, 91, 132;   *see also* clinics
   storage   39, 60, 65
factories   19, 21, 71, 89, 101, 102101
faecal-oral   15, 28, 29, 31, 42
falciparum   100;   *see also* malaria
family   15-21, 26, 30, 36, 37, 39-41, 43, 49, 50, 51, 55, 57, 58, 60, 73, 74, 81, 83, 84, 90, 100, 126, 128
farmer   15, 19, 28, 49-52, 54-60, 102
FAO (food and agriculture organization)   57
fever   105, 126
filters   111
fertile   30, 63
fertility rate   13, 15, 16, 89, 90, 130;   *see also* TFR
fertilizer   21, 28, 51, 52, 54-58, 60
fire   40, 56, 97
firewood   56, 58
fishing   49
flour   71
food and agriculture organization;   *see* FAO
foodstuffs   40, 43, 52
foraging   49

forests   57, 58
freshwater   29, 57
fruits   38, 42, 60
fuel   39-41, 44, 51, 56, 67, 68, 70 ,72
fuelwood   41, 55, 58

G
garden   57, 60
gardening   49
gawan   53, 54;   *see also* caag
goitre   37;   *see also* deficiency, iodine
gonorrhoea   18;   *see also* STD
grain   52, 59, 69, 70, 71
green manuring   56
grinding   71
growth   36, 38, 52, 53, 94
guinea worm   30

H
H. influenza   96, 97
Hackett's spleen class   113, 114
haematuria   30, 110, 111, 132
haemoglobin   36, 100, 111
Haemophilus   97
haemoptysis   126
harvest   50, 51, 53, 56, 59, 71
harvesting   49, 51, 58, 59, 60, 72
heart disease   103
halo effect   29
hand-washing 27, 28, 42
health
    centre   83, 85, 91;   *see also* clinic and facilities, health
    survey   7, 8, 35, 64, 123, 131, 133
height   100, 101
helminthiasis   14
hepatitis   112
herd immunity   98
high-risk   13, 35, 38, 79, 88, 101, 131, 132
HIV   18, 103
horse   70
hospital   10, 14, 70, 84, 86, 95, 97, 126
hot/cold theory   43
hunting   49
hybrid   51, 52
hydroelectric   71
hygiene/hygienic   27-29, 31, 95, 97
hypertension   110
hypothyroid   36

I

immunization   83, 87, 90, 97, 98, 103, 123, 124
immunized   63, 90, 97, 98
income   13, 16, 18-20, 26, 30, 39, 40, 49, 66, 70, 73-75, 81, 83, 85, 87, 90, 100
India   11, 16, 18, 35
infant mortality   16, 18, 92
infanticide   18
infections   18, 29-31, 37-39, 93, 94, 98, 99, 108, 111-113
    respiratory   94-97
infectious   25, 29, 35, 39, 40, 82, 92, 93, 98, 104, 112
infertility   18
injuries   21
insects   44, 59, 60
intercropping   56
intrauterine growth retardation;   *see* IUGR
iodine deficiency   36
iron   55, 58
iron deficiency   36
irrigation   51, 52, 54, 58, 60
IUGR (intrauterine growth retardation)   36

J

K

kala-azar   112
kerosene   72;   *see also* paraffin
key informant   82, 130-133
kitchen   40, 42, 91
kwashiorkor   16; *see also* PEM

L

land   18, 20, 41, 49, 50, 51, 53-55, 57, 58, 60, 73, 88, 100
larvae   30, 44
latrine   28, 29, 57, 65
laundry   29
leader   6-8, 63, 91
legumes   41, 43
leguminous   56, 57
leishmaniasis   14
leopard skin   104, 108, 109
leprosy   104, 107
Leucaena   56
Liberia   8, 43, 66, 102
lifestyle   79, 101, 103
literacy rate   13, 20
literate   64, 105, 126, 129

literature   53, 73, 88, 91, 99, 102
   published   8, 9, 79, 80, 87, 97, 99, 105, 126
   searches   9, 21, 105
loan   50, 75
low birthweight   37, 94, 97, 98
lymph nodes   108
lymphadenitis   107

M

machinery   51, 69, 71, 74
maize   52, 56
malaria   14, 30, 31, 54, 81, 82, 95, 98-101, 105, 107, 111-113, 130
maldistribution   94
malnourished   68, 93, 94, 97, 104
malnutrition   1, 16, 18, 28, 35, 37-39, 43, 44, 49, 93-95, 97, 100, 112
mammals   59
manganese   55
mango   44
manure   57
masons   63
maternal child health;   *see* MCH
maternal depletion syndrome   16, 17
maternal mortality ratio;   *see* MMR
Mazotti reaction   108
MCH (maternal child health)   88
meal   27, 28, 38, 39, 41, 43, 69
measles   14, 94, 97, 109, 112, 123
meat   42
medicine   1, 65, 75, 84-87, 96, 105
menarche   128, 129
merchants   55
microfilaria   108, 109;   *see also* onchocerciasis
microscope   107, 108, 111, 112
mill   69, 71
millet   52
milling   59, 69
minerals   60
ministry of health   9, 10, 87, 97
MMR (maternal mortality ratio)   88, 89, 127, 130
mobility   100
money   19, 40, 44, 50, 72-76, 85-87, 123, 130
morbidity   25, 27, 30, 31, 37, 38, 73, 88, 92, 93, 97, 99, 100, 103, 104, 109-111, 132
mortality   13, 14, 16, 18, 31, 37, 38, 73, 92-94, 96, 97, 99, 100, 102-104, 109, 111, 127-130
mosquito   30, 99
multimixes   41-43
Muslim   84
myalgias   105

N

need, perceived   81-83
neonatal tetanus   90
NGO (non-governmental organization)   9, 10, 75
Niger   80, 87, 92, 94, 95
night blindness   109, 110; *see also* xerophthalmia
nitrogen   55-57
nitrogen-fixing bacteria   56
non-governmental organization; *see* NGO
NPK fertilizer   55
nutrient/s   38, 54-58
nutrition   1, 16-18, 20, 28, 35-38, 40-44, 50, 60, 94, 97

O

observation   1, 4, 7, 10, 11, 21, 29, 30, 81, 82, 84, 87, 91, 101, 107, 126
occupation   21, 101, 102
occupational injuries   20, 21, 101, 102
oil   43, 58, 112
onchocercomata   107
onchocerciasis   30, 101, 104, 107-109
oral rehydration
    solution   96, 97
    therapy   95, 96
oranges   44
organophosphate   102
overcrowding   97
ox   73

P

panhandling   103
paraffin   72
parasitic   30, 31, 82, 92
pawpaw   44
Peace Corps   10
PEM (protein energy malnutrition)   97, 112; *see also* kwashiorkor
penicillin   85
pepper   43
pertussis   97
pesticide   21, 102, 103
pests   15, 59
petrol   67, 68, 70
pharmaceutical   83, 85
PHC (primary health care)   1, 5, 76, 84
phosphorus   55
photovoltaic   71
placenta previa   36
planting   53, 56, 59
plumbers   63

pneumonia   85, 96, 126
poisoning   55, 102, 103
polio   107
pollution   14, 21, 97, 101
population   1, 8, 10, 13, 16, 20, 27, 31-32, 49, 50, 52, 54, 58, 60, 64, 80, 81, 83, 87, 89, 91, 95-98, 100, 108-110, 114, 123, 124, 127-133
   density 14, 15, 18, 83, 123-124
potassium   55
potato   38, 52
pots   39, 41, 42, 44
pregnancy   14, 16, 35, 37, 127-130
pregnant   14, 35, 43, 84, 98, 99, 128
premature, death   35, 36, 92, 95, 100
prematurity   94
preservation   42
prevalence   6, 14, 18, 30, 31, 36, 81, 89, 90, 94, 97-99, 104, 106-109, 111, 112, 123, 125, 127, 130-133
primary health care;   *see* PHC
private voluntary organization;   *see* PVO
prostitution   103
protein   39, 43, 44
protein energy malnutrition;   *see* PEM, kwashiorkor
proteinuria   110, 111
pruritis   108
pulmonary   40
pumps   26, 28, 53, 71
PVO (private voluntary organization)   9, 10, 75

Q
questionnaire   125-127, 130-133

R
rain   29, 52-54
rainy season   6, 25, 53, 55, 99
random sampling   124, 125
REA (rapid epidemiological assessment)   4, 123, 133, 134
recall bias   126, 128
refrigeration   39, 42
refrigerators   70-72
reservoir   26
respiratory   82, 94-97, 101;   *see also* ARI
resources   2, 4, 6, 7, 9, 10, 13, 14, 16, 17, 19, 20, 38, 50, 55, 58, 63, 64, 68, 72-75, 78, 79, 82, 83, 86, 88, 89, 100, 102, 103, 104, 107, 110, 111, 114, 123, 127, 133
revolving drug fund   86, 87
rice   31, 38, 43, 52, 54, 59, 99
river   26, 30, 58, 69, 71
river blindness   101, 107;   *see also* onchocerciasis

roads   55, 65, 67, 69
rodents   59, 60

S

S. pneumonia   96
salting   42
sample size   110, 124, 125, 128
sampling
    cluster   123-125, 133
    random   123-125
sanitary   42
sanitation   10, 14, 31, 95
scale   35
schistosomiasis   29-31, 54, 110-112, 130-133
Schistosoma haemotobium   105, 110, 111, 130
screening   2, 30, 108-110
scurvy   44
seed   51, 52, 58, 60
services   10, 13-15, 50, 64, 74, 79-85, 87, 92
sexually transmitted disease; *see* STD
shortage   26, 27, 39, 41, 43, 50, 56, 58, 72, 85, 87, 95
Simulium black fly   30
sisterhood method   127-130, 136
skin snips   108
slaves   50
slums   14, 15, 26
smallpox   123
smoke   40
smoking   42, 97, 103
snail   29
soil   52-54, 56-58
solar   53, 57, 71, 72
sorghum   52
soy beans   56
spleen rate   99, 112-114
splenomegaly   105, 111, 112, 114
staple   15, 38, 41, 43, 50
statistics   1, 9, 10, 13, 21, 58, 73, 80, 81, 88, 91, 101
STD (sexually transmitted disease)   18, 103
stealing   103
steel   66
stillbirth   36
stool   28, 57, 105
storage   26, 39, 41, 42, 49-53, 58-60, 65, 71
stove   40, 56, 65, 67
stovepipe   40
stream/s   25, 28, 53, 54, 71, 101
street children   103
stroke   103

stunting/stunted   35, 36
subsidized 83
surgical   85
survey   3, 6-9, 11, 19, 22, 31, 35, 44, 64, 81, 82, 97, 105, 107, 109, 114, 123, 127, 130, 131, 133, 134, 137
swamp/s   99, 101
swimming   29

T

TALC (Teaching Aids at Low Cost) 76, 95
TB (tuberculosis) 14, 97, 104, 107, 126
TBA (traditional birth attendant) 91
technology   60, 69
termite   44, 65
terracing   53
tetanus   88, 90
TFR (total fertility rate)   89
thatch   66
thresh   59
thresher   69
timber   57
tobacco   97
toilets 29
traditional healers   64, 65, 80, 83, 84
transport   14, 19, 39, 67, 102
transportation   14, 50, 55, 67-69, 84, 85
trauma   101
trees   56, 58, 102
tropical ulcers   104, 107
truck   67
turbines   71
typhoid   112

U

ulcers   30, 104, 107
undernutrition   35, 50, 53, 93, 94, 100, 112
underweight   35, 37, 94
unemployment   19
UNICEF   9, 76
urbanization   17, 18, 37, 90, 103
urine   28, 29, 105, 111
　　filtration   110, 130, 131, 132
　　reagent dip sticks   110, 111, 131, 132
USAID   9, 75
utensils   39, 41, 42
utilization 81-84

V

vaccination   87, 90, 97, 98, 123
vaccine   72, 95, 97, 98
vaccine refrigerator   70-72
vector/s   29, 42
vegetables   38, 42, 43, 60
vehicle/s   20, 55, 67
verbal autopsy   125-127, 133
vertical programmes   87, 96, 97
violence   93
Vitamin A   60, 94, 97, 109, 110
vitamins   60
vote   88

W

walking   44, 68
wasted   2, 9, 10, 36, 59, 104
water   1, 7, 14, 15, 25-31, 49, 52-54, 58, 66, 69-71, 85, 95, 99, 132
    collection   25, 28
    container   26
    piped   26
    quality   25
    quantity   25, 27, 28
    scarcity   26
waterwheels   71
wealth/y   10, 50, 54, 107
weaning   17, 37-39, 41
weight   35, 37, 94, 95, 100, 101, 126
wells   25, 26, 29, 53
wheat   52
WHO   1, 5, 9, 37, 76, 85, 88, 97, 102, 105, 110
wind   53, 70, 71
windmill   71
women   6, 11, 14-20, 28, 35, 37, 39, 41, 43, 50, 51, 69, 79, 84, 88-91, 98, 99, 103, 128, 129
wood   41, 58, 65, 66

X

xerophthalmia   109, 110
xerosis   109
X-rays   70

Y

yams   38, 52
yield   30, 49, 50, 51, 52, 54, 55, 57, 58
yogurt   42

Z

zinc   55